Chronic Pain Gone 90 Days

How to eliminate the pain of
  Arthritis
  Headaches
  Fibromyalgia
  Back pain
  Neck pain
  Joint pain
  Carpal tunnel syndrome
  Sciatica
  Digestive upset

  by finding the cause and eliminating it

Dr. Daniel A. Twogood

Printed in the United States of America

Published by
Wilhelmina Books
Apple Valley, California

ISBN Number 978-0-9631125-4-5

Library of Congress Control Number: 2011936398

Dedicated to Bill Green

July 29, 1935 - November 10, 2010

A fellow truth seeker

Chronic

It lasts a really long time.

It is not going to go away.

The doctor has advised you to:
Learn to live with it.

Pain

Discomfort that means something is wrong.

Tissue damage is happening, or is going to happen.

It's a pain.

Gone

The pain went away.
Learn to live without it.

90 Days

The chain of events that take place

when healing begins *and is unimpeded*

will end chronic pain in 90 days.

How to Use This Book

This part of the book is an instruction manual about how to get rid of chronic pain.

This part of the book is unreferenced.

You can go to the library or the internet and find lots of studies that **support** the information you are about to read.

Those studies don't matter.

You can also find lots of studies that **refute** the information you are about to read.

Those studies don't matter either.

This book is based on my many years of practice, practicing to find what works in the **elimination** of pain.

Not the *treatment* of pain. Lots of people are doing that.

I've learned a thing or two while practicing on people.

These are my observations.

If you suffer with chronic pain, you've been to doctors who have practiced on you.

But here you are.

Here is another approach that your doctors have not tried.

The fastest way to get results with this book is to skip to page 9, read the names of the 10 chapters (ingredients), then do what the chapters say.

Do that for 90 days and you will have completed your own study.

And only one study matters.

Only your study matters.

This study has produced excellent results for many people.

Many of those people had no hope.

There is always hope.

I hope you have the same experience.

If you follow the instructions in this book, you will know if the information is valid or not.

For you.

This program is rote.

Please don't over-think it.

Save your mental energy for fortitude, because success will depend on it.

Please don't mix in any conventional medical folklore.

You don't have to do anything extra to succeed. In fact, if you do nothing, that will be more successful in eliminating pain than *doing* anything else.

This program requires *not* doing certain things.

I have tried to use as few words as possible.

If you want more words, turn to page 45 and read the pages that follow, or use that part for a reference.

The chapters are listed from one to ten in order of importance, like the ingredients list on a package of processed food.

The first ingredient on an ingredients list occupies the highest percentage of stuff in the container — there's a teeny bit of the last ingredient.

The first chapter is the most important instruction, and so on down the list.

You may eliminate your chronic pain by doing only the first and second chapters, or maybe three or four.

The best chance of eliminating chronic pain is accomplished by doing the entire list for 90 days.

If you want to know what to do, right now, without wasting any more time, skip to page 9, read it, and follow those instructions for 90 days starting right now.

Or, just do this and you can be done immediately:

For the next 90 days, swallow only these things: fruits, vegetables, rice, beans, eggs, oatmeal, grits, unsalted nuts, pure meat, and water.

No supplements are necessary. Save your money.

For a better understanding of *why* you are doing this, read the rest of the book.

Modern medicine is ineffective in eliminating chronic pain.

You know this to be true.

In fact, if modern medicine worked for your condition, it was not chronic pain, and you wouldn't be reading this book.

This program is very simple.

This program is not easy, but it is simple.

Part One: Ingredients

1. Do It Now

Don't *try* these instructions.

People who are *trying* to quit smoking, or *trying* to get some exercise, are still smoking and not exercising.

Trying = not doing it.

Don't try.

Do it now.

Exercise programs don't work.

Diet programs don't work.

This program doesn't work.

They only work if you work.

Don't do it tomorrow.

Don't do it next week.

Don't start after you use up all of your bad food.

This is the first chapter and the most important.

You can start now and continue reading.

The following instructions mean nothing, unless you

do it now.

2. Don't Eat Casein

Casein is found in **dairy foods**, and many non-dairy foods.

Dairy foods are made from cow's milk.

All foods made from, or made with cow's milk, contain casein. (goat's milk also contains casein)

Casein is the most common cause of pain.

All foods are made of protein, fat, and carbohydrate.

The fat and carbohydrate portion of milk are not factors in pain.

Butter is milk fat and has no casein.

(Skim milk and low fat milk contain casein)

The protein faction of milk is made up of three main proteins:

Casein

Lactoalbumin

Lactoglobulin

The last two proteins make up whey.

Reactions to whey are very rare.

The carbohydrate portion of milk is **lactose.**

Lactose intolerance is digestive upset caused by lactose.

Most digestive upset is lactose intolerance

Lactose intolerance and casein allergic reactions are not related.

You can have one without the other.

Lactose free milk (Lactaid™) contains casein and must be avoided.

Many *non dairy* foods contain casein.

Foods that contain caseinate cause pain.

Sodium caseinate, calcium caseinate, any kind of caseinate causes pain.

Most coffee creamers, like Cremora™ and Coffeemate™ contain casein in the form of **sodium caseinate.**

Flavored coffee creamers contain caseinate.

Ensure™ contains caseinate.

Cool Whip™ contains caseinate.

Many protein shakes contain caseinate.

Caseinate must be avoided to eliminate pain.

The most common food allergen is casein.

Most **headaches** are reactions to casein.

Most **back pain** is caused by casein.

Most **arthritis** is caused by casein.

Rhematoid arthritis is allergy — usually to casein.

Nerve pain is caused by casein (sciatica, carpal tunnel).

Recurrent ear infections in children is allergy to casein.

Asthma is allergy — usually to casein.

12

Streptococcal infections will not occur in children who consume no casein.

Growing pains — milk allergy.

Bed wetting is allergy — usually to casein.

Fibromyalgia is allergy — usually to casein.

Other Reactions to Casein

Carpal Tunnel Syndrome

Sciatica

Half head headache

Most headaches

A knot, or a burning pain under the shoulder blade

Joint pain

Muscle and joint stiffness

Nasal drip and congestion

Muscle stiffness

Leg cramps

Frequent urination

Many skin reactions are allergy to casein, like:

Psoriasis

Eczema

Acne

Most acne is allergy to casein.

Female problems are often due to casein:

Infertility

Ovarian Cysts

Endometriosis

Varicose veins

Miscarriages

Many behavioral problems are due to casein:

Attention deficit

Hyperactivity

Depression

Schizophrenia

Crepitus (joint noises, like cracking, popping): casein.

Allergic reactions can be **mild:**

    red cheeks in kids
    crepitus
    lethargy

to **severe,**

    anaphylaxis
    SIDS (sudden infant death syndrome).

To avoid all casein, avoid all foods made from or containing animal milk or any form of casein or caseinate:

DO NOT EAT

Whole Milk

Low Fat Milk

2% Milk

Non Fat Milk

Skim Milk

Buttermilk

Cheese

Cottage Cheese

Ice Cream

Ice Milk

Sherbet

Ranch dressing

Caesar Dressing

Bleu Cheese

Sour Cream

Cream Cheese

Pizza

Whipped Cream

Egg Nog

Canned Milk

Parmesan Cheese

Yogurt

Also avoid caseinate in:

Coffee Creamers

Soy Cheese

IMO™

Cool Whip™

Protein shakes

I Can't Believe it's Not Butter ™

Ensure™

Mayonnaise, butter, and eggs contain no casein.

3.   Chocolate

Never, ever, eat it.

Chocolate is the most powerful cause of pain.

Even the smallest amount of chocolate can cause a severe reaction.

All people who react to casein in milk and dairy foods also react to chocolate....

...only the reaction is worse...

Even chocolate that contains no milk.

Even artificial chocolate.

Even chocolate flavoring.

Eat no chocolate candy bars, hot chocolate, Ovaltine™, cookies, ice cream, chocolate soy milk, chocolate protein shakes, etc.

18

Chocolate can cause:

Back pain

Neck pain

Joint pain

Headaches

Nerve reactions like:
- Depression
- Irritability
- Anxiety
- Carpal tunnel
- Sciatic pain
- PMS

Many women crave chocolate around the time of their menstrual cycle.

Many of these women suffer, along with their families, with PMS symptoms.

Many PMS symptoms are caused by chocolate.

If you suffer with any kind of chronic pain, eating chocolate will make it worse.

4.   Eat No Processed Foods
(Mainly to avoid MSG)

Processed foods contain many chemical substances that are poisonous, harmful, or questionable.

Many processed foods contain Monosodium Glutamate (MSG) or Aspartame

MSG and aspartame are nerve toxins that can cause pain.

Monosodium Glutamate (MSG)

MSG is found in many spices, processed meats, TV dinners, canned and dried soups, restaurant soup, breaded foods, flavored snack foods, and sauces (BBQ, soy sauce, teriyaki, Worcestershire, etc.).

Pure spices (salt, pepper, fennel, cumin, etc.) contain no MSG....

....except **MSG** or **Accent**™ which each contain only one ingredient: **monosodium glutamate**.

Spices that are mixtures of spices, like lemon pepper, taco seasoning, Italian seasoning, etc., often contain MSG.

Mrs. Dash™ **products contain NO MSG.**

Most restaurants use some MSG.

Many restaurants use lots of MSG (see chapter 7, "Don't Eat Restaurant Food")

Food manufacturers hide MSG under other names, like:

20

Hydrolyzed proteins

Yeast extract and autolyzed yeast

Natural flavors

Flavoring

Spices

Protein isolate (found in most protein shakes)

Some of these ingredients may contain MSG, and maybe they don't.

Ground beef in fast food tacos contains autolyzed yeast.

If a food product says **"No MSG"** there is a good chance that is true.

Any food that says **"No MSG Added"** contains MSG.

Any restaurant that claims they don't **add** MSG, uses MSG.

Any claim of "No MSG†," is a lie. That product contains MSG.

Look down to find the * or † that says, "except for that which is naturally occurring in yeast extract."

It's in really small print. (see page 167, 168)

Vegetarian meats and meals made with Textured Vegetable Protein (TVP) contain MSG.

Strictly avoiding foods that contain MSG and aspartame will be essential for recovering from chronic pain.

Monosodium glutamate and aspartame are known to cause and contribute to pain and chronic pain.

To avoid these chemicals, it is not necessary to avoid all processed foods with labels, but that would be a very good way of doing it.

To be sure, avoid all foods that have a list of ingredients.

MSG is a flavor enhancer.

MSG is a nerve toxin.

MSG is toxic to the nervous system.

MSG irritates the nerve endings on the tongue (taste buds) causing them to respond more powerfully, sending a message to the brain that is interpreted as saltier, or beefier, or more sour....yummier.

The flavor enhancement is often described as

Fuller flavor

Spicier

Bolder taste

Zestier

Toxins are dose dependant, like alcohol:

Small amount = small reaction
Large amount = large reaction

Small doses day after day will increase the dose and will cause a more severe reaction.

MSG irritates the taste buds on the tongue so food tastes better.

But after MSG is swallowed it makes its way into the blood stream where it causes symptoms through nerve irritation.

In small doses MSG causes symptoms in sensitive people.

In large doses MSG causes symptoms in **all** people.

Common symptoms of MSG exposure are:

Mood changes
Heart palpitations
Panic attacks
Heart attacks
Shortness of breath
Fullness in the throat
Pain (75% of the time on the left side)
Headaches
Swelling in the hands
Carpal tunnel syndrome
Mysterious bruises (the size of a dime)

Some reactions don't cause symptoms until much later, after many years of exposure.

Neurological symptoms like dementia, Alzheimers, Parkinsons, and other forms of neurological degeneration can be caused by MSG and other nerve toxins, like alcohol and aspartame.

The most common reaction to MSG looks like a heart attack:

> Chest pain
>
> Shortness of breath
>
> Left arm pain
>
> Panic
>
> Musculoskeletal pain (left side 75% of the time)

MSG causes many heart attacks.

Many processed foods contain MSG.

MSG is one of the most powerful causes of pain.

To eliminate chronic pain, all MSG, in all of its forms, must be eliminated.

If you avoid processed foods and restaurant food, you will avoid MSG.

Aspartame

Aspartame is found in diet foods and sodas, most chewing gum, sugar free foods, and artificial sweeteners (**Equal and Nutrisweet**).

Aspartame is also a neurotoxin. Aspartame is chemically similar to MSG. Aspartame stimulates the sweet taste buds and gives the illusion of sweetness.

MSG and aspartame have no taste.

The taste sensations caused by MSG and aspartame are hallucinations.

MSG does not stimulate the sweet taste buds, so it is not used in pastries, fruit drinks, candies, and other sweet foods.

Aspartame is used in nearly all chewing gum.

Most diet and low sugar foods contain aspartame.

If it is too difficult to read labels searching for these substances,

avoid all foods that have a label.

Avoid foods that are processed in such a way that artificial substances are added to the final product.

Many food additives are unhealthy, some are dangerous, and some are "generally regarded as safe" by the FDA.

Some are nerve toxins, like aspartame and MSG.

Some are carcinogenic, like nitrates and nitrites found in processed meats, like any tubular meat (sausage, hot dogs, chorizo, kobassa) and deli meats (salami, bologna, turkey loafs, ham loafs, etc.).

Others are questionable, like butylated hydroxytoluene (BHT), and butylated hydroxyanisole (BHA) used in cereals.

Sodium pyrophosphate, carrageenan, maltodextrin, and thousands of others are questionable substances that do not contribute to your well being.

To end chronic pain, all processed foods must be avoided.

Protein shakes are unhealthy.

5. Just Say No to Drugs

Always say no to cholesterol drugs.

All drugs are poison.

All drugs cause effects **and** side effects.

Some people need drugs. Those include:

> People with genetic diseases like hemophilia, and type I diabetes.
>
> People who have taken a drug for many years and whose bodies have come to rely on them.
>
> People who are unwilling to change their diets and lifestyles.

Most people who take drugs don't need them.

If you are not yet using prescription drugs, thank goodness.

Don't start down that road. It will lead to poor health and a premature and miserable death.

If you currently take prescription drugs, your body may have come to rely on them, and quitting will be difficult.

Continue taking your prescription drugs for 90 days, then hopefully, you can quit......

Except for statins for cholesterol.

If you are taking a cholesterol pill, quit it immediately.

Best selling pill of all time:

Vicodin for pain.

Vicodin relieves pain sometimes.

Second best selling pill in the world:

Lipitor for cholesterol.

Lipitor causes pain sometimes.

Lipitor is a statin drug used to lower cholesterol, other statins are:

Zocor, vytorin, pravachol, symvastatin, Crestor, mevachor

Gemfibrozil and zetia cause the same symptoms.

Leg and foot weakness, numbness, cramps and back pain are common symptoms caused by cholesterol drugs.

Very common.

Doctors will tell you that high cholesterol causes an increased risk of heart attack and strokes.

Statins **do** lower your cholesterol (too much).

Statins **do not** reduce your risk of heart attack or stroke.

Statins **can** cause liver damage and muscle pain.

Do not ever take statin drugs, or any cholesterol pill.

If you have unbearable pain, and you take a pill that eliminates the pain, that is a good pill — for now.

It's a good pill to take until you heal.

But the long term use of anti-inflammatory drugs will cause an elevated level of inflammation, and more pain.

The longer you take any pill, the more likely you are to suffer side effects.

Blood pressure pills, cholesterol pills, and many others change your blood test scores, your report card.

Your doctor is happier, but you're not.

Drugs are toxic substances that unbalance an already unbalanced system.

An unhealthy system (your body in pain or disease) is rebalanced best by subtracting, not adding.

Is there a pill, a cough suppressant, that will stop the cough of a smoker?

Sure. But it makes more sense to subtract the cause of the cough than it does to suppress a cough that is functional.

Smoke and tar and nicotine being sucked into the lungs need to be expelled.

Cough, cough, cough, hack, hack, hack, until you quit smoking. No pill needed.

Subtract, don't add.

Don't start down the medication path to poor health.

Just say no to drugs.

6.   Don't Eat Gluten (wheat)

Gluten is the main protein in wheat.

Gluten is also found in barley, rye, spelt, and semolina.

Gluten is found in :

    Bread (white, wheat, rye, potato, sour dough, etc.)
    Crackers
    Cakes
    Cookies
    Pasta
    Breading
    Flour tortillas
    Most cereals
    Pretzels

Gluten is an allergen that causes reactions in people who are sensitive to it.

After casein, gluten is the most common food allergen.

Many people are allergic to gluten.

People who are sensitive to gluten are usually sensitive to casein.

Common reactions are:

Pain

Nerve irritation

Digestive upset (Crohn's, IBS, diarrhea, constipation, GERD).

Most digestive upset is caused by dairy foods and/or wheat.

Nerve irritation can include:

    Pain

    Sciatic pain

    Carpal tunnel syndrome

    Headaches

    Mood changes (like depression, schizophrenia, bipolar disorder)

    Neurofunk (puzzling disorders like multiple sclerosis,Huntington's Chorea, Dementia, Alzheimer's, paresthesias and neuropathy)

Any allergen or toxin can cause any or all of the above.

Why is gluten a common allergen?

Casein is found in cow's milk. Cow's milk is a natural food for baby cows and is not healthy for humans. Makes sense.

But wheat is the staff of life, right?

The original wheat from Mesopotamia was good for humans.

But wheat has been changed many times. It was cross-bred and hybridized many times over the centuries.

And then in the 1950's Norman Borlaug won the Nobel Prize for changing wheat into a crop that saved millions of starving lives.

He changed wheat by exposing wheat seeds to radiation, causing mutations that led to a species that was hardier and more productive.

Many people were saved. But some people cannot tolerate the new strain, and that's called:

Gluten intolerance.

Gluten intolerance is now so common that all health food stores and many grocery stores offer gluten-free foods.

Starchy alternatives to gluten include:

> Gluten-free breads and pasta
> Rice flour pasta
> Potato chips
> Corn chips
> Corn tortillas
> Rice Chex™ Cereal
> Corn Flakes or grits
> Oat cereal or oatmeal

Gluten intolerance can also cause digestive upset, often called celiac disease.

Whether it's Irritable Bowel Syndrome (IBS), diarrhea, Crohn's Disease, Colitis, most digestive upset is caused by gluten, dairy foods, and/or medication.

Gluten is a common cause of chronic pain.

7. Don't Eat Restaurant Food
(mainly to avoid MSG)

Restaurant food is processed food.

Most restaurants use some MSG, and some use lots.

Many will claim "No MSG," which is not always true.

Some say "No MSG Added" which means they serve foods that already contain MSG.

Sauces (like teriyaki, BBQ, soy, au jus, etc.) are used for flavor, and most of them contain the most common and powerful flavor enhancer, MSG.

Ground beef in fast food tacos contains autolyzed yeast.

Soups in restaurants usually contain MSG.

Salad dressings usually contain some MSG.

Most breaded foods contain MSG and gluten and dairy.

Steaks are often treated with MSG.

You just don't know what is in all those tasty foods.

It's just too risky to eat foods prepared by others until after your ninety days is up.

Later, after you have recovered, you can experiment with restaurants to find out where you can eat and not react with pain or other problems.

But for now, it's best to prepare your own food.

8.   Move Your Body - a lot

I know a lot of you young folks want to run really far and fast and build a body that looks really hot.

But that's not necessary to eliminate or avoid chronic pain.

To avoid chronic pain you just have to keep moving.

You have to practice moving every day in the directions and the ranges of motion that are necessary for life.

You have to move almost all the time.

Don't just sit or stand or lay there.

Move. More is better.

Adhesions (cob webs) form in your joints within minutes.

If you are inflamed by one of the aforementioned allergens or toxins, these adhesions hurt when you finally get moving and they tear loose.

Immobility aggravates chronic pain.

Sleeping is eight hours of immobility and leads to stiffness.

Stiffness leads to pain

Sitting puts a lot of pressure on your lower back.

So does standing in one place.

So move.

Exercise: Experts will tell you there are right and wrong ways to exercise. I agree.

The right way — exercising the way you like.

The wrong way — not exercising.

1. You must **walk**.
> You need to walk to enjoy life the best way possible.
> Keep walking and you can always walk.

2. You must be able to **get up**:
> Out of bed
> Out of a chair
> Up off the ground if you fall.

3. You have to **reach** things that are up high.

4. You have to **reach the floor** to pick things up.

5. You have to be able to **look all around**, up, down, and
> sideways:
> to see where you are going.
> to see what's coming at you.

When you can't, you will need a care giver.

Do this every day to avoid and eliminate chronic pain:

1. Walk three miles every day.

("I walk around a lot at home or at work" doesn't count.)

Walk three miles without doing anything else.

More if you want.
(If your pain prohibits this, wait until you're better)

2. Reach up as high as you can with both hands, then bend over and touch your toes.

Do this ten times in the morning, and ten times at night.

More if you want.

3. Squat down, sit on the floor. Then lie on your back on the floor. Look at the sky or the ceiling.

Then get up the best way you know how.

Do that three times a day.

More if you like.

4. Stand up, look up, look down, look to the right, look to the left, touch your left ear to your left shoulder, then your right.

Do that three times each day.

More if you like.

5. Be as tall as you can at all times, while sitting or standing.

9. Eat Only These Foods

Fruits

Vegetables

Rice

Rice flour pasta

Beans

Eggs

Unsalted nuts

Pure meats

Corn chips (unflavored)

Potato chips (unflavored)

Oatmeal

Grits

Drink Only:

Water

Herbal Tea

Fruit juices

Plant based milks (soy, rice, almond, coconut)

10. No Smoking

Sucking smoke into your lungs screws everything up. You don't get enough oxygen, so later on you have to carry it around in a bottle.

When you don't get enough oxygen, your healing mechanism doesn't work properly.

In 1994 the tobacco industry had to reveal the chemical content of cigarettes. They listed 599 substances, most of which cannot be pronounced.

Cigarettes contain chocolate (the most powerful cause of pain), hydrolyzed milk solids (casein and free glutamate, MSG), and lots of other stuff that is no good for you.

It says right on the package that cigarettes are harmful to your health and can cause cancer and emphysema.

Any substance besides clean air sucked into the lungs is hazardous to your health, including second-hand smoke, smoke from fires, marijuana, crack, huffing, etc.

Smoking will not help you heal from chronic pain.

So please, don't smoke.

*The Good News

You don't have to do this forever.

If you have managed to follow the previous ten steps for ninety days, you are indeed disciplined.

And you should feel much better.

To continue forever avoiding dairy, chocolate, processed foods, MSG, restaurant foods, gluten, and all drugs forever would be next to impossible. It would be best, but very difficult and may make you unhappy.

The good news is that you probably don't have to be so strict forever.

This is for two reasons:

1. Your chronic pain is probably caused by only one allergen or toxin.

2. Your sensitivities may decline the longer you avoid the particular allergen or toxin that affects you.

Most chronic pain is caused by casein in dairy foods.

You may be able to avoid chronic pain the rest of your life by just avoiding dairy foods, and eating anything and everything else you want......

Except chocolate.

Every person who reacts to dairy foods also reacts to chocolate, only worse.

Most chronic pain is solved by eliminating all dairy foods and chocolate. Gluten and medications are less common as causes of chronic pain.

If your chronic pain is caused by gluten, then casein and chocolate will also cause inflammation.

Most people can remain free of chronic pain by reverting to a diet that looks more like moderation — controlled moderation.

Controlled moderation is also called a rotation diet.

When an allergen is avoided for 90 days, most people will experience a decreased sensitivity to it.

After 90 days of avoidance, the allergen will still cause a reaction, but the reaction will not cause noticeable symptoms … in most cases.

It takes about a week for an allergen to be consumed and make its way through the system.

If your first exposure to casein after 90 days causes no reaction, you are among the 80% of chronic pain sufferers who will be able to consume casein…

…no more than once a week.

One exposure to an allergen will cause an increased inflammatory reaction for 3, 4, or 5 days, up to a week.

After 90 days, exposure to the allergen should be limited to once a week. That will allow the inflammation to abate.

All drugs are poison.

A second dose within a few days will cause the piggyback effect: one dose plus another (before the inflammation dies out) could cause symptoms.

To be safe, limit exposure to two times a month.

Twenty percent of people with a casein sensitivity have a fixed allergy: they will react each and every time they are exposed to the allergen.

Remember *the phenomenon of changing symptoms:* you could have a new reaction to the allergen (page 129).

Toxic substances, like nicotine, alcohol, carbon monoxide, caffeine, MSG, aspartame, and drugs are dose dependant.

You may not have a noticeable reaction to a toxin (or an allergen). But the ongoing, sub-clinical inflammation may cause tissue changes and damage to tissue that may not cause problems until it is too late to reverse the damage.

All medication is poison, and long term use of any medication will eventually cause side effects.

Never take statin drugs.

More good news:

You can return to restaurants as you figure out which ones, and which dishes, don't have MSG, and how to avoid casein, or gluten, or just the one or two substances that bother you.

Let's all have fun once in a while, have a goody now and then, eat out when you want.

But remember what you learned in your study here, and realize that allergies are not outgrown, and poison is poison and always will be.

Part Two: More Information

1.   What Causes Chronic Pain?

This book is about pain, and how to eliminate it. Specifically, it's about chronic pain, pain that doesn't go away, or keeps coming back for weeks and weeks and years and years.

It is not difficult to understand the pain that happens after you stub your toe or bonk your head or hit your thumb with a hammer.

In these instances, you realize that a physical event applied too much stress to a body part, and it hurt. Maybe it bruised or bled. You may be upset, but you are not puzzled. You are not going to read a book about that kind of pain.

You know that the pain is going to go away in a reasonable period of time. You are not going to the doctor. You can treat it at home with ice or drugs or cursing or rubbing it or by just doing nothing until it goes away.

Your body heals.

But chronic pain is different.

Your body fails to heal.

In many cases of chronic pain, the sufferer can remember a physically stressful event, an auto accident, a fall, years of physical labor, etc. that seemingly caused the pain.

Sometimes chronic pain sufferers can't remember a specific event, and many times the physically stressful event isn't all that stressful. Some people claim they slept wrong. Their pain happened in bed, and they were alone.

In many cases the chronic pain is the same recurring problem that keeps coming back for no apparent reason. Doctors and patients all study that one spot, the lower back, that bad knee, he neck, those headaches, that numbness in the hands, sciatic pain, weakness in the legs, those symptoms that keep coming back, or just won't go away.

In other cases it is a migrating pain. One day it's under your shoulder blade on the right, the next day it moves to the left.

The assumption is that the damage done by some physically stressful event caused irreversible damage. You assume it's irreversible, or chronic, because you've tried everything to no avail. You just haven't healed.

Doctors will prescribe lots of tests and lots of drugs, but there is usually no good explanation for your lack of healing. X-rays are usually negative.

MRI's are expensive and almost never change your treatment program.

It's just drugs and tests, over and over again.

The questions that must be answered are:

What is interfering with the normal healing process?

What makes the pain keep coming back?

What can be done to promote healing?

Instead of answering these questions, doctors are probing the exact location of the pain to find out what is wrong with some specific tissue. Is it a ligament? Is it a muscle? Nerve?

Then they can name it, like fibromyalgia.

Trying to determine which specific body part is involved is pointless.

Even with multiple opinions, and after waiting for definitive tests that never are, eventually therapists soldier on with some sort of treatment.

You've tried chiropractic care, physical therapy, drugs, supplements, rest, heat, ice, and pain management. Maybe even surgery. Maybe several surgeries. You've worn braces.

The people who had good results with those therapies are not reading this book. They're better already.

All of these techniques work to a certain degree.

But you and I both know that there are many people who are still suffering despite lots of treatment, tests, and diagnoses. Many people are resting at home on disability. They don't go to work anymore. They are suffering financially and emotionally. Yet they still have pain. They are not healing despite the fact that they have eliminated the physical stress that seemingly caused their pain.

Many of you have tried lots of medications. Some of them work for a while. Then they stop working. You try other pills. You suffer with the side effects, yet your pain remains. The pills may mask the pain, but without them, the pain comes back.

Pills are not healing your chronic pain.

Some people have had surgeries. Several surgeries. They still have pain. So it's called chronic.

Physical therapy and chiropractic care offer some relief. But you have to keep going and going or the pain comes back. It's like bailing water out of a leaky boat. It works great until you stop.

It seems that chronic pain requires chronic treatment. You don't buy one pill, you get a big bottle, and you have to keep renewing your prescription until you are addicted or you get an ulcer or your insurance decides they won't pay for that pill, you have to switch.

The notion that physical stress causes physical pain is obvious. You bonked your head too hard, or you stubbed your toe too hard, or you worked at that job too long. You have felt pain many times in your life.

The first thing you experienced was a slap on the butt to make you cry. We have all been programmed to look at chronic pain in the same way we look at regular pain: it's a physical phenomenon.

People who suffer with chronic pain, and doctors, are stuck in this mind set that all pain is physical. To treat it you must rub it, or immobilize it, or stretch it, apply heat, or maybe ice, or maybe both, cast it, brace it, bolt it together, remove it, shave it, manipulate it, etc.

But many people who suffer with chronic pain know that their history is not all that physically traumatic. Or they've been convinced that minor activities like typing and walking have caused their pain.

Rheumatoid arthritis is extremely painful, but most sufferers know that it wasn't physical wear and tear that caused their gnarled, bent, and painful joints.

Certainly physical activity aggravates arthritis, but those who suffer with arthritis are usually no more physically stressed than people who don't have arthritis.

And even if it was physical stress that caused your pain, why haven't you healed? Why doesn't rest help? Why doesn't the pain go away when you have stopped working?

Physical stress does not cause chronic pain.

Physical stress may *aggravate* chronic pain.

Chronic pain seems to be caused by lots of factors. Pain is caused by the accumulation of many forms of stress. You have noticed your chronic pain is affected by the weather, by the time of year, by your state of mind, your diet, your genetic makeup, the traffic conditions, the rotation of the earth, the moon, etc.

Chronic pain is a puzzlement in many cases, and many sufferers are constantly trying to guess as to why they felt bad one day and good the next or vice versa.

Some cases are very, very complicated, and some of you may not find the solutions in this book.

But most cases of chronic pain are solved very simply.

The only way to solve chronic pain is to determine it's cause, then eliminate it.

X-Rays and MRI's are over-rated and over used.

2. Pain is Caused by Too Much Stress

Definition: **Stress** is *any* stimulus that elicits a response.

Stress is life and living. Life without stress is no life.

Even while you are sleeping, you experience the physical pressure of the sheets and blankets, you feel the rise and fall of your breathing, the beating of your heart, the response to your dreams.

Without some stress, there is no life. A fulfilling life includes stress, and your response to it.

Stress is stimulating.

But *too much* stress is painful.

If a person rubs against you, they have applied physical stress to your body. It doesn't cause pain.

A masseuse applies physical stress to your body. It doesn't hurt, well except for that deep tissue torture. A massage is physical stress, but it feels good.

If you get slugged in the face it hurts. Getting slugged is too much physical stress.

Jumping down off of a curb is stressful, but usually not too much.

Jumping off a two-story building is too much stress. It hurts.

Stress comes in three forms:

> **Physical stress**
> **Mental stress**
> **Chemical stress**

Chronic pain is caused by the accumulation of these three forms of stress.

Getting a massage is a form of physical stress.
Getting run over by a car is too much physical stress.......pain.

Solving a difficult math problem is mentally stressful.
The death of a loved one is too much mental stress.......pain.

Drinking one cocktail is a form of chemical stress.
Drinking too much alcohol is too much chemical stress....pain.

Chronic pain is caused by the accumulation of all forms of stress. Trying to determine what is the cause of the pain you are feeling right now, pain you didn't have when you went to bed last night, is very difficult when you don't consider all of the factors, all of the stressors that could have contributed to how you feel.

Was it something you did two days ago? A week ago? Was it that accident you had years ago? Why were you ok yesterday, and now you're in killer pain? Did you sleep wrong?

When you consider only the physical stressors, the answer to what is causing your chronic pain is elusive.

But remember, chronic pain is not caused by physical stress.

Chronic pain may be aggravated by physical stress, but not caused by it.

Jeff looks like Santa Claus in overalls, a dirty old baseball cap, and tiny bifocal glasses. He collects junk in Barstow. Each day he hooks up his mule to his old wooden buckboard wagon and cruises town picking up junk.

One day he picks up an old refrigerator, some luggage, a bunch of books, tools, scrap metal, some used carpet, and lots of other stuff.

After a few hours his wagon is full and creaking, so he heads home to his two-acre junkyard.

Just around the corner from home he comes across an old abandoned bicycle. He picks it up and tosses it on top of his load and the wagon breaks.

Jeff says the bicycle broke his wagon.

But was it just the bicycle that did his wagon in?

In order to fix the wagon, he will have to unload all of the junk, not just the bicycle.

Hans Selye

The definitive work on stress was done back in the early 1900's by Hans Selye and is explained in his book, *The Stress of Life*.

Hans Selye was a medical doctor who was born in Vienna in 1907 and educated in Europe. He performed his world famous research in Canada.

While he was a medical student and was studying the various signs and symptoms of specific diseases, he noticed that most diseases shared many of the same symptoms. Fever, aches and pains, weakness, rashes, sinus congestion, stomach upset, headaches, etc.

This observation made him think: maybe there is a disease that is *just being sick in general.*

While specific germs, allergens, and poisons cause specific symptoms, many of the symptoms are the same.

Selye began experiments with rats by torturing them and eventually killing them, then performing autopsies on them.

He tortured the rats by exposing them to the various forms of stress.

One group of rats was caged in a cold environment (physical stress).

Another group was injected with a slow acting poison (chemical stress). (like smoking or the Standard American Diet)

And another group was mentally stressed by having their legs tightly bound to their bodies (mental stress).

All three groups were fed and watered regularly, as was a control group.

All of the rats exposed to the three forms of stress became sick and eventually died.

But Hans Selye noticed that each group of rats had the exact same response, even though the forms of stress were different.

At first, the rats became sick and lost weight. Then they seemed to adapt for a period of time, even though the stressor was still being applied. Their weight leveled out. But later, as the stress continued, they lost more weight and their health deteriorated until they died.

Selye performed autopsies on these unfortunate rats.

All of the rats had the same autopsy results:

> enlarged adrenal glands
>
> atrophy of lymphatic tissue
>
> gastrointestinal ulcers

And all of the rats arrived at their deaths through the same series of events. No matter what form of stress was applied, the response was the same.

Selye called the whole process the *generalized adaptation syndrome.* Internally, the response involved hormone and other chemical changes in the blood. The response was generalized no matter what form of stress was applied, and it was adaptive: it led to healing, unless the stress was overwhelming.

Overwhelming stress leads to chronic pain and then to an uncomfortable death.

The Generalized Adaptation Syndrome

As stress is applied, the body goes through a three phase response:

The Alarm Reaction

The Stage of Resistance

The Stage of Exhaustion

In cases of acute pain, the sensation of pain is part of the alarm reaction. Many other microscopic changes take place that lead to healing.

The body produces both pro-inflammatory and anti-inflammatory substances that course through the blood stream and control the stage of resistance and lead to healing.

Pain and swelling are part of the normal response and are essential for the healing process to be completed successfully. These are pro-inflammatory reactions. The body produces and circulates specific substances that lead to pain and swelling.

All pain is caused by inflammation.

The introduction of anti-inflammatory medication and pain pills interrupts this normal process.

The long term use of drugs does more to contribute to chronic pain than it does to eliminating it.

The chronic use of anti-inflammatory drugs to treat chronic pain will cause an increased pro-inflammatory condition (increased pain and swelling) that builds up between doses of the anti-inflammatory.

The anti-inflammatory drug (naprosyn, ibuprofen, motrin, aspirin, alleve, advil, etc.) will lower the level of inflammation and pain. But when the drug wears off, the level of inflammation will rebound to a higher level. The decrease in pain that results from the pill will be followed by an increase in pain as the drug wears off, causing the chronic condition to become more painful over time.

Pretty soon you are taking a handful of pills every day just to feel lousy.

The treatment for all pain and disease is the same:

The natural healing mechanisms of the body must be allowed to proceed unimpeded.

Acute pain goes away when the cause of the inflammation is stopped or removed.

Stop hitting your thumb with that hammer and it will heal and the pain will go away.

Chronic pain persists because the cause of inflammation has not been removed.

The solution to chronic pain is to remove interference with the healing system, not in attempting to amplify the healing mechanism with drugs or supplements.

Drugs like vicodin, darvocet, codeine, oxycontin, or percoset dull your brain's perception of pain, but they do not stop the source of the pain.

The stressors that are causing pain must all (or mostly) be eliminated in order for healing to proceed.

The presence of stressors to the body impede the healing process and must be eliminated in order for the pain to go away.

It's not just the last event, the last straw, or the biggest event that causes chronic pain.

It wasn't just the bicycle that broke Jeff's wagon.

Jeff can't fix his wagon by just removing the bicycle or the fridge.

He has to unload the wagon completely (or at least mostly) to fix it.

When pain becomes chronic, the stressors have not been removed. If you quit working and stop lifting in an attempt to eliminate the stress, and your pain does not go away, you have not eliminated enough of the stressors that are contributing to your pain.

At this point, most patients and doctors become resigned to the notion that you are not going to get better. You must "learn to live with your pain."

Your condition is called **chronic = no hope.**

But there is always hope.

When you systematically remove each form of stress for long enough, your body will heal and pain will go away.

All pain and all disease is caused by the **accumulation** of the three forms of stress:

    Mental stress
    Physical stress
    Chemical stress

Mental Stress contributes to chronic pain very minimally. While many people believe that mental stress is the main cause of pain and disease, that isn't true.

Your mental state can certainly contribute to and detract from your health, but you don't have to believe that a poison will kill you for that poison to kill you. If you don't believe that poison will kill you, it will anyways.

You can use mental fortitude to act sober when you are drunk, but the booze wins, no matter how strong you are mentally.

A positive attitude contributes to health and happiness and goes a long ways to fighting off pain and disease. That kind of attitude, and the ability to successfully manage mental stress can provide the fine- tuning in solving chronic pain issues.

While many people jump to the conclusion that the word stress implies mental stress, **stress is applied in a more harmful way physically and chemically.** If you have a bright and sunny outlook on life and are able to let troubles roll off your shoulders, it won't help that much if you smoke and drink, eat unhealthy foods, take drugs, and participate in dangerous activities.

A positive attitude always helps some, but not when physical and chemical stressors are overwhelming.

Physical Stress can be applied all at once, like falling off a cliff. Physical stress can also be applied a little at a time, over days and years, like repetitive motion disorders (stuffing envelopes all day).

A shoelace won't break the first time you tie your shoes. But eventually it will break. It wasn't the first tug, or the last. It was the accumulation of all of the repeated tugging that eventually caused the lace to snap.

Sitting at a typewriter and typing 100 words per minute doesn't require much movement as far as range of motion is concerned. But typing for hours may cause your fingers to cramp up or get stiff and sore. Typing every day for years and years can certainly cause chronic problems.

For every job that requires physical stress (every job), there are good and bad ways to perform those duties. Ergonomics has become very popular, especially in the last few years. Work stations are analyzed and changed to accommodate workers and their activities in an attempt to decrease the amount of physical stress that may contribute to pain and disability (and worker's comp claims).

Typewriters used to be manual and required much more power to push the keys. Electronic and digital typewriters, computers and calculators require much less strength and pressure to operate. Some are now voice activated.

Over time, shovels and hoes and the sweat and toil of thousands of men have been replaced by modern equipment that requires far less sweat and toil and wear and tear and pain. The manual and hydraulic levers on earth moving equipment have been replaced by joy sticks. With these innovations, huge amounts of rock and dirt can be moved with the flick of the wrist.

Eliminating the physical stress that contributes to chronic pain involves avoiding too much physical stress, and preparing the body to handle physical stress with exercises that enhance strength and flexibility.

Reducing physical stress is an important part of eliminating chronic pain.

But Chronic Pain is caused by chemical stress.

Chemical stress is the most powerful contributor to chronic pain and disease. The human body is equipped with an amazing healing mechanism that is moderated through the body's chemistry. Chemical stress interrupts this mechanism and prevents healing, causing chronic pain.

Chemical stress is caused by exposure to:

> toxins
> allergens
> germs

Germs can be handled by a healthy immune system that is not compromised by allergens and toxins. We are exposed to germs every day, and we handle them, every day.

Allergens and toxins cause chronic pain.

When the normal chemical functions of the body are interrupted, or enhanced, or changed in any way, problems will eventually occur.

While conventional medicine continually insists that changing the body's chemistry through the liberal use of pharmaceuticals is the way to treat chronic pain, they are wrong.

Drugs that lower blood pressure, or cholesterol, or the inflammatory response, or drugs that interfere with calcium metabolism to supposedly build stronger bones, drugs that depress your nervous system so much that you fall asleep instead of worrying, or don't give a hoot instead of worrying, all of these pills that doctors insist are necessary for health are toxic substances that mask symptoms and cause more health problems than they solve.

Some pills are the cause of chronic pain.

But if you feel bad, and you take a pill that makes you feel good, or better, that can be a good thing once in a while.

But when your problem is chronic, using poisonous drugs on a regular basis will lead to major health problems. And that's the problem with the modern medical system that allows pharmaceutical companies to apply their profit motive to the health care system in such a powerful way that **American medicine has become what it is:**

Largely ineffective and often downright dangerous.

Drugs are poison.

Poisons are dose dependent.

You may not notice any reaction to a small dose of poison. You will feel a bigger dose, get sick with yet more, and if you get enough of a poison, you will die.

Alcohol is poison:

> One drink may make you happy.

> > With three or four you may get lucky.

> > > College binge drinking will kill you.

Poisons can have their effect from one big dose, or many smaller doses applied over time. An alcoholic is poisoning himself on a regular basis, and he will go through life like Hans Selye's rats:

Alarm reaction (drunkenness),

Period of adaptation (hung-over, but able to go to work)

Exhaustion: liver failure and death.

The body is able to handle a dose of poison once in a while, but long term exposure will eventually overwhelm the body and lead to exhaustion.

Healthcare for profit aims to get more and more people to take the drugs that are prescribed for a lifetime. Lifetime prescriptions are huge doses of poison that will eventually cause pain and disease.

Witness many of our elder citizens who are taking drugs for blood pressure and cholesterol and their various aches and pains and their impending osteoporosis.

They're a mess. They are demonstrating the end of their ability to adapt and the beginning of their exhaustion. They shake, they're weak, they're befuddled — they are exhausted and about to be extinguished — by their medication.

A pill that makes you feel good is one thing. But when a doctor prescribes a pill that merely changes your report card (blood test) and you still feel bad, what is the point? Pharmaceutical companies aspire to create drugs that MUST be taken forever. Or you will die, they say.

Even a handy little aspirin, good for headaches and pain and such, has been relegated to the "once every day" category. That s what people have come to believe, that you need it to prevent heart disease — it's good for you.

But check out the bruised and bloody forearms of old people who have taken aspirin every day.

Aspirin is not good for you. It's poison.

This book is an instructional manual on how to eliminate chronic pain by making simple changes that remove the interference to healing.

The most powerful affect on the human condition is in controlling the blood chemistry.

The blood chemistry is affected by what we eat, inhale, inject, and absorb through the skin.

Our most intimate contact with substances that either nourish us or poison us is in what we swallow — diet and medication.

Making the changes necessary to eliminate chronic pain involves changing what you allow into your digestive tract.

Substances that you swallow make their way into your blood stream.

That is the foundation of modern medicine. When you consult a doctor for almost any condition, you will most likely be given a prescription for some chemical concoction that you are instructed to swallow on a regular basis, for several days, weeks, or maybe even forever.

To a certain degree, everything you swallow either nourishes you or poisons you.

Every substance contributes to your health, or to your lack of health.

Every substance you swallow helps to eliminate chronic pain or contributes to chronic pain.

This program involves making specific changes to your diet and medications.

While many professionals and supplement manufacturers and pharmaceutical companies claim to have developed their own unique magic concoction that will cure all your ills, this program is about elimination, not addition.

There's nothing to be bought or sold here.

This program requires no supplements. You don't have to purchase expensive vitamins or protein shakes. In fact, it's better if you avoid these products.

You don't have to shop for exotic foods in health food stores. In fact, it's better if you stay out of health food stores, except for the few (very few) natural foods that you can't find in any regular grocery store. Unless you just want to pay more.

You don't have to join a gym to get rid of chronic pain.

You don't have to purchase special equipment to eliminate chronic pain.

You don't need health insurance to eliminate chronic pain.

Staying away from doctors will help more than sitting in their waiting rooms too long for the little bit of time they spend with you to tell you what some drug rep told them to say.

Conventional medicine is ineffective when it comes to treating chronic pain successfully.

Conventional medicine is largely ineffective for two reasons:

1. Doctors rely on drugs as their main tool.
2. Doctors almost never consider the diet.

Almost no doctor will consider diet changes to treat pain, but it seems the diet is important when the patient has high cholesterol, heart disease, or digestive upset. In these cases I've asked patients if their doctors discussed their diets. The answer is usually "no", but some say the doctor told them to watch what they eat.

What does that mean? When I ask the patients that question, they usually respond, "You know, no greasy food, stuff like that."

Chronic pain comes from within the body, not from the outside. Even conventional doctors have realized that the most powerful way to affect the human condition is by changing the internal environment, changing the blood chemistry.

A chemical substance is placed in the mouth, inhaled, or injected into the skin and it makes it's way into the blood stream.

The blood carries the substance everywhere in the body and it has an effect. Blood pressure pills like lisinopril and atenelol and hydrochlorothyazide block certain cardiac functions and the blood pressure is lowered.

You don't need doctors to eliminate chronic pain.

Anti-inflammatory drugs like motrin, advil, alleve, naprosyn, celebrex, and ibuprofen inhibit certain parts of the inflammatory reaction, decreasing inflammation and pain.

Recreational drugs go through the same process. They are inhaled or swallowed or injected, they get into the blood stream, and they have an effect.

While conventional medics realize that changing the blood chemistry can be used to treat the human condition, they have failed to realize that it is changes in the blood chemistry that *cause* most pain and disease.

Our most intimate contact with chemical substances that change the blood chemistry, and therefore affect the human condition, is what we eat, drink, and swallow.

The diet has the most powerful affect on the human condition.

I take that back. The diet has the *second* most powerful affect on the human condition. Most people are shy or outgoing, big, fat, or small, clear skinned or not, left or right handed, blue or brown eyed, or have a tendency for cancer or heart disease or pain, because of their **genetic makeup**.

We are hard-wired to be who and how we are. We cannot change that. We all know people who smoke and drink and eat bad food and live to be 100. Good genes.

Bob Hope and George Burns, smokers and drinkers, both outlived Jack Lalanne.

If you want to change your size or shape or how you feel, you have to change your diet. More specifically, if you want to change, you have to change what you put into your body.

Chronic pain has a cause.

It's not what you did.

It's what you ate.

You have to change what you allow to get into your blood stream.

To a certain degree, everything you allow into your blood stream will either nourish or poison you.

Everything you allow into your blood stream will either contribute to your health, or take away from it.

Everything you allow into your blood stream will contribute to pain, or contribute to healing.

This book is about how to eliminate chronic pain. There is certainly a pure, perfect diet that is best for everyone and will solve most health problems.

3. Dairy Foods Cause Most Chronic Pain

Casein, one of the proteins in cow's milk and cow milk products, is the most common cause of chronic pain, arthritis, fibromyalgia, and headaches.

Many doctors and government agencies have told us for years that milk is essential for health. Strong bones and no osteoporosis will be the result of consuming milk and dairy foods regularly. Without milk, they say, we will all wither up and die.

This is not true.

Many other researchers and practitioners have written about milk and it's contribution to disease processes.

Marshall Mandell, M.D. wrote a book in 1975 about the relationship between food and disease. The forward to that book was written by **Abram Hoffer, M.D.**, a psychiatrist. This is what he wrote:

Over the years I began to accumulate a substantial number of chronic patients who had not responded adequately. They did not recover. About five years ago I became more and more concerned about this group. I became aware of the work being done by Dr. Mandell and Dr. William Philpott, an orthomolecular psychiatrist. I saw a film Dr. Mandell had made at one of our meetings. My interest gradually arose. What deterred me was that I knew so little about food allergies and how they were investigated. Eventually I was forced to become involved by my patients.

*A sixteen year old **schizophrenic** girl had not responded to any treatment given by her psychiatrist, then by me. One day I realized that nothing was working and she was doomed to become a **chronic**, hopelessly ill schizophrenic. This motivated* *me to act. I persuaded her to fast for four days. On the fourth day she was normal. This I had never seen in over twenty years of practice. She was allergic to milk and a number of other foods.*

A glass of milk reactivated her psychosis in an hour.

Over the next two years I made about 160 patients fast. About 100 responded in the same way. This work has been corroborated by other orthomolecular psychiatrists. There is no further doubt in my mind that certain peoples' brains react adversely to a variety of substances by becoming schizophrenic. If cerebral allergy can cause that most deadly of all mental illnesses — schizophrenia — it can surely mimic all the other conditions as well, such as learning and behavior disorders, depression, anxiety, etc., and it does.

Robert Foreman, Ph.D. wrote a similar book in 1984, *How to Control Your Allergies.* On the second page of his book he wrote the following, the first case study in his book:

A colleague of mine recently underwent about $700 of diagnostic tests as medical school doctors tried to locate the cause of a variety of symptoms, including muscle pains, digestive upset so severe they woke him up in the middle of the night, and a feeling of weakness and lack of energy. They mentioned the possibility of various uncommon scary diseases but could find nothing conclusive. When, at my suggestion, he tried experimenting with his diet to see if foods played a part, he quickly found that **all his troubles came from a sensitivity to milk,** *which he of course then stopped drinking.*

One day shortly after this he popped his head into my office to tell me, 'I was able to ride my bicycle today for the first time in more than a year.' And another time he stopped by gleefully reporting, 'I painted my garage over the weekend. A few weeks ago I could barely hold a brush.'

Jethro Kloss wrote the classic **Back to Eden** in 1939. The only mention of milk in his 600 page book is as follows:

Cow's milk is not suited for human consumption. Half the invalids in the world suffer from dyspepsia, and milk should not be taken. Milk causes constipation, biliousness, coated tongue, headache, and these are the symptoms of auto-intoxication. Soybean milk, and nut milks are excellent substitutes, and have practically the same analysis; and the danger of disease is removed.

John McDougall, M.D. has been giving out some of the best diet information for many years. He calls dairy foods *"the most harmful of the traditional four food groups."*

He goes on to say:

"Dairy products are also the leading source of food allergy, causing a wide range of problems from headaches to bed wetting, stuffy nose, and even death."

Kurt Oster, M.D., and Donald J. Ross, Ph.D. wrote the **XO Factor** and had this to say about milk and heart disease:

The malignant influence of continuous homogenized milk intake containing biologically active xanthine oxidase is, in my opinion, a greater health evil than cigarettes.

Frank Oski, M.D. was the head of pediatrics at Johns Hopkins University School of Medicine and Physician in Chief of the Johns Hopkins Children's Center when he wrote **Don't Drink Your Milk**, his book about childhood illnesses caused by milk, like recurrent ear infections and bed wetting.

Check out **Robert Cohen's** 1997 book, **Milk The Deadly Poison.**

Dr. Daniel Twogood has been saying the following for 25 years:

Most chronic pain is caused by dairy products.

Most people who suffer with chronic pain could stop right here — just eliminate all milk and dairy foods, and chronic pain will be eliminated within 90 days, probably sooner.

Cow's milk is specifically designed to be the perfect nutrient for a growing calf. An analysis of all the milk of the different mammals, horses, goats, humans, dogs, cats, mice, whales, etc., shows that they are all quite different, each suitable for their own newborns.

Milk, like every other food, is made up of protein, fat, and carbohydrate.

Most digestive upset is caused by lactose, the carbohydrate portion of dairy foods. Most people who suffer with gas, bloating, constipation, diarrhea, irritable bowel syndrome, Crohn's disease, GERD, and ulcers, would get great relief by eliminating dairy foods.

Even the dairy industry is pushing non-fat and low fat products because of the unhealthy animal fat in their products.

Cow milk protein is made up of three proteins: lactoalbumin, lactoglobulin, and casein.

Casein is the protein that causes the inflammatory reaction that is milk allergy.

Pain is caused by an inflammatory reaction set off by casein, the main protein in cow's milk, and all foods made from cow's milk, and many non-dairy foods that contain casein in the form of sodium caseinate, or calcium caseinate, or any form of caseinate.

Caseinate is found in processed foods, especially so-called non-dairy foods like coffee creamers, soy cheeses, Cool Whip™, Ensure™, protein shakes, and some margarines (I Can't Believe it's not Butter™ contains caseinate). The symptoms of milk allergy will be set off by non-dairy foods that contain casein.

The inflammatory reaction is an allergic reaction, and can affect any tissue.

Skin reactions include eczema, psoriasis, and acne.

The reaction can take place in the tendons, joints, muscles, in the blood vessels, or in the nervous system.

The chronic, continuous use of dairy foods is the most common cause of chronic, ongoing inflammation that is called chronic pain.

Many cases of acute pain are caused by casein. Especially when pain comes on for no apparent reason, or after some minor physical activity, chemical stress is the most likely cause.

Casein is the most likely culprit.

The pain caused by inflammation as a reaction to ingested casein in dairy foods can come on instantaneously, or as long as 48 hours later.

The most common reaction time is 2 to 12 hours.

Each inflammatory reaction lasts for 3, 4, or 5 days, and can last up to a week.

Allergic reactions are not dose dependant. If you have a sensitivity to casein, it doesn't matter how much you have, it's how often you have some.

A little cream in your coffee daily is a regular dose that can cause chronic pain.

Non-dairy creamers (especially the flavored ones) containing caseinate are very powerful at causing nerve pain and muscle and joint aches and pains.

When casein is completely eliminated, chronic pain due to casein (most cases) will disappear within 90 days.

Casein in dairy foods is the most common cause of pain.

Dairy foods include:

All animal milk (whole, Vitamin D, skim, 1%, 2%, non-fat, butter milk)
Goat milk
Cheese
Cottage cheese
Yogurt
Sour Cream
Cream cheese
Ice cream
Ice milk
Sherbet
Pizza
Ranch Dressing
Bleu Cheese
Feta
Parmesan cheese

Caseinate is found in:
Coffee Creamers
Protein Shakes
IMO™
Cool Whip™
I Can't Believe It's Not Butter™
Some Soy Milks
Many processed foods and meats (salami)

All people who react to dairy foods in a bad way also react to chocolate — but the reaction is worse.

Chocolate is the most powerful cause of pain.

Even chocolate that contains no milk, like cocoa, will cause pain.

Even artificial chocolate, like in Oreos™ and other foods that contain chocolate flavoring will cause pain.

Rheumatoid arthritis and Fibromyalgia are usually caused by dairy foods.

Lupus erythematosis is allergy — usually to casein.

However, other chapters in this book explain that other allergens and toxins can cause the same reactions.

Symptoms

The most common cause of ongoing chronic pain is the casein in milk and dairy foods.

Recurrent ear infections in infants and toddlers is milk allergy. (Gluten may also cause ear infections)

Most kids outgrow ear infections, even when they continue to drink milk. **There are two reasons for this:**

1. Babies look like little space creatures because they have big heads and little faces. The cranium grows first and fastest, and the jaw and lower face grow a little later. When the jaw and lower face are smaller in the first few months and years of life, the Eustachian tubes (from the ears to the oral cavity) are horizontal. When the baby is upright, or lying down, the tubes do not drain. There is no downhill. Any mucous production in the Eustachian tubes from an allergen stays in the tubes, clogs the tubes, and bacteria grow, causing ear infections.

As the child ages, the face elongates and the tubes drain downhill into the oral cavity. If the child continues to eat dairy foods, the allergen (casein) causes the production of mucous that drains into the mouth where the slimy bacterial concoction then causes tonsillitis and strep throat infections. When it drains into the lungs, the poor little guys cough and cough and cough — called the croup or bronchitis.

Allergy to casein in infants who are nursing is made possible by a mom who ingests dairy foods.

Many baby formulas contain milk and casein or caseinate.

2. Tissue adapts to the ongoing onslaught of an allergen or a toxin. It adapts, or bucks up. The alarm reaction becomes the period of adaptation. But if exposure to the allergen continues, the affect will show up in other tissue (see the Phenomenon of Changing Symptoms, coming up shortly). The mucous production will occur in other tissue, and other "itis's" will be the result:

dermatitis, laryngitis, arthritis, colitis, bronchitis, etc.

Streptococcal bacteria live in the mucous membranes lining the airways and the mouth and nasal passages. Their populations explode when allergic mucous is produced, providing a nice environment for the germs. Sickness ensues, sore throats, tonsillitis, colds, coughs, etc.

In Frank Oski's book, ***Don't Drink Your Milk***, Dr. Dan Bagget, M.D., a pediatrician has noticed, and says,

"Streptococcus germ will not, under ordinary circumstances, establish an infection in a child kept on an absolutely no-milk-protein dietary regimen."

Tonsillitis, sore throats, bronchitis, and ear infections are caused by casein.

This should be common knowledge among pediatricians. But pediatricians prescribe drugs for these kids, then put tubes in their ears, and almost never consider the diet.

Bed-wetting is milk allergy and all pediatricians should know that too.

Bet you never heard that one from a doctor. One of my patients didn't believe me until he read it in *Reader's Digest*.

For years parents and doctors have considered that bed-wetting is a psychological problem, and bad parenting is the cause.

81

Many parents have pulled their hair out for years fearing such a notion is true. They parented three or four other kids in the same way, but those kids didn't wet the bed.

Don't punish a bed wetter. Take dairy foods out of the diet. Problem solved.

Growing pains is a weird diagnosis. There is no pain involved with growing. That's just when it's happening, and there seems to be no other explanation. There's no other explanation as long as diet changes are not considered.

These nebulous pains in the legs and joints and muscles and back that cause kids to cry is not imagined.

Growing pains are milk allergy.

Inflammation is caused by casein and often manifests itself as pain that can't be explained, or pain that can't be explained logically, like severe back pain that resulted from sleeping wrong.

Adolescent diseases caused by casein include asthma and acne.

Asthma is inflammation of the airways caused by allergic inflammation.

Many people assume that inflammation in the airway is caused only by inhaled substances like cigarette smoke, smog, dust, pollen, mold, and perfumes and animal dander.

Inhaled irritants can indeed aggravate the airways, but most cases of asthma are caused by ingested allergens.

Allergy testing is often inconclusive, and allergy shots don't help. Steroidal inhalers are prescribed. Steroidal inhalers are over-prescribed. Too many kids are using albuterol and other inhalers that can cause weight gain and other side effects.

Most asthma is caused by dairy foods, animal dander, and MSG (monosodium glutamate).

Acne is inflammation of the skin pores caused by casein in dairy foods.

Many of these symptoms seem to be outgrown even when the children continue to eat dairy foods. But symptoms change with time, they don't go away.

Allergies are not outgrown.

In his research on stress, Hans Selye discovered that stressed animals get sick at first, but eventually settle into a period of adaptation. The symptoms seem to go away even though the stressor is still present.

When the damaged tissue is able to adapt for a long enough period of time, that tissue will heal. But eventually another body part or system will fail and become diseased, or distressed...there will be new symptoms.

I call this the **Phenomenon of Changing Symptoms**.

Susan came into my office at the age of twenty-one complaining of neck and shoulder pain and headaches. She was a regular dairy user so I discussed the diet changes that would be necessary for her recovery.

She told me she "used to be allergic to dairy foods" at age 15 when her face would swell up and her eyes would swell shut. At that time doctors had no answers other than steroids. But she and her mother figured it out. Each time she ate a dairy food, her face swelled up within 30 minutes. So she quit dairy foods and all was well until at age 19 she got married and began eating dairy foods again. Since her face didn't swell up, she thought she was over the milk allergy.

Her headaches and neck pain were caused by casein. These symptoms were eliminated after she stopped eating dairy foods. Again.

Allergies are not outgrown. They do not go away. Specific symptoms may change, but there will always be an inflammatory response once the allergy has been established. The inflammatory response may be sub-clinical. The inflammation may begin in an organ that is so healthy that it will take a while to show symptoms.

One such organ is the substantia nigra, an area of the brain composed of billions of nerve cells that control fine motor movements. If that organ is affected by an allergen or a toxin, it will take many years before symptoms of Parkinson's Disease become apparent.

But once enough of the cells are destroyed by the inflammatory process, the shaking will begin and continue to get worse.

Alzheimer's disease is another example of neurological degeneration over time that only becomes apparent when enough neural tissue is destroyed by the inflammatory reaction to allergens and/or toxins.

The nervous system is highly susceptible to damage done by allergens and toxins. Alcohol (a toxin) causes the immediate reaction of drunkenness. But with heavy use over time, alcohol will actually liquify the nerves, leading to the psychoses and other phenomena associated with alcoholism: confabulation, bad behavior, family destruction, drunk driving tragedies, child abuse, spousal abuse, a negative perception of reality, sex between unlikely partners, and jobs for overweight bouncers.

Multiple Sclerosis (MS) is another neurological disease where parts of nerve cells become hardened, interrupting nerve conduction, therefore causing the neuro-funk of the disease.

The sclerotic areas are caused by recurring inflammation and repair caused by long-term exposure to an allergen or a toxin.

Multiple sclerosis can be caused by casein or gluten.

It is the ongoing inflammation, repair, and scarring of any and all tissue that causes the many, many symptoms of chronic pain and disease.

Chronic exposure to allergens and toxins, diet and medication, are the cause of chronic disease.

Most of this destruction is caused by casein in dairy foods.

In adults, the most common reactions to casein are:

neck and back pain and stiffness
headaches
shoulder blade pain
joint pain
stomach upset
sinus problems
heart conditions
sciatic nerve pain
carpal tunnel syndrome
frequent urination
varicose veins

Pain in the muscles and joints has been classified ad-nauseum by anyone, trained or otherwise, anyone who has an opinion.

The different diagnoses for pain don't matter.

All that matters is that you have pain, and the naming and classifying and imaging of that pain doesn't change a thing.

MRI's, CT Scans, and x-rays are over rated. They don't change your condition.

Chronic neck pain, back pain, joint pain, nerve pain, headaches, fibromyalgia, and arthritis are caused by allergens and/or toxins.

Inflammatory reactions to dairy foods are caused mainly by casein. But there are other factors in cow's milk that cause reactions.

The Cholesterol Myth

Robert Ester told me his story in 1985 and I didn't believe him. He told me how he suffered with chronic pain and headaches for twenty years. He consulted all kinds of doctors and therapists to no avail. His condition got worse and worse until he was unable to work.

The doctors he consulted for many years had lots of ideas about what he should do, in their expert opinions, about his condition. None of it worked.

Acupuncturists, chiropractors, orthopedists, neurologists, internists and psychiatrists all took stabs at solving his chronic pain, unsuccessfully.

He tried acupuncture and massage and lots of different pills.

He had tests and more tests. Several doctors told him he had high cholesterol, 285, and that he would die if he didn't take medication. Even though he chose to *not* take their drugs, he was scared. He gave up on his chronic back pain, but decided to attack the cholesterol issue by doing his own research and acting on his own. He changed his diet and began walking three miles a day. He went back for re-testing in three months. He had lost twenty pounds and his cholesterol had dropped to 185.

He was also pain free.

He went back to work.

After a while, he began missing the foods he had eliminated to lower his cholesterol. To lower his cholesterol, he eliminated all foods that contain cholesterol, which is all animal foods: all meats, eggs from chickens, and dairy foods from cows. He did this for six months and felt fine, no pain.

After six months, he missed meat, so he started adding it back into his diet. He had no problems. He added eggs back into his diet. No problems.

But every time he tried to eat a dairy food, his back went out and he got a migraine.

I didn't believe him.

He told me neither did any of his doctors.

I researched his claim and found nothing in the literature.

A few months later, I began experimenting with diet changes in difficult cases. I saw results right away, luckily, and wrote my first book, *No Milk*, in 1991.

But let's get back to cholesterol. It's a common notion that elevated cholesterol is caused by eating too much cholesterol. This is not true.

Cholesterol is produced by the human body and pumped into the blood stream to repair damaged arteries. Arteries are damaged by inflammation. Inflammation in arteries is caused by circulating toxins and/or allergens.

The chemicals in cigarette smoke cause lots of problems, including inflamed arteries, high blood pressure, elevated cholesterol, and heart disease.

But most arterial inflammation is caused by xanthine oxidase, an enzyme that is biologically active in homogenized milk products.

Xanthine oxidase is found inside the cell membrane of the fat globules in cow's milk. When milk is not homogenized, like in raw milk, the fat globules are large and are broken down by digestive enzymes in the intestines. The xanthine oxidase is exposed and destroyed in the intestines.

The fat globules of homogenized milk are much smaller after they have been forced through fine screens. The fat globules in homogenized milk are suspended in milk uniformly. These small fat globules are absorbed by the intestines whole and protect the xanthine oxidase from destruction in the intestines. In the blood stream, xanthine oxidase eats holes in the arterial walls.

The body responds by increasing circulating cholesterol.

Lowering cholesterol with statin drugs (lipitor, zocor, mevachor, pravachol, crestor, symvastatin, vytorin, and others) is a mistake. A huge mistake. These drugs remove the fire trucks without addressing the fire — the inflammation.

The drugs used to lower cholesterol are not harmless candy. You will read in chapter ten that statin drugs are extremely harmful, causing liver damage, kidney damage, and chronic pain in the form of leg weakness and pain, back pain, sciatic pain, and all over the body pain and weakness.

The most effective way to lower cholesterol is to:

1. Stop smoking

2. Eliminate all dairy foods (casein and xanthine oxidase)

3. Increase cardiovascular activity.

What about osteoporosis?

Many times in distance running events at track meets, one team will send out a "rabbit" to set the pace. The rabbit is on pace to shatter the world record, but we all know what is going to happen. The other runners run a faster race trying to keep pace with the rabbit. But well before the finish line, the rabbit is exhausted. The field passes him up and he finishes last, or doesn't finish at all.

Life is like that. We are trying to get to the end without running out of energy, vitality, or money.

Excessive exercising will speed up the using-up of muscle cells. Huge bulky muscles won't be that way when you're seventy.

Excessive exposure to the sun (and tanning beds) speeds up the using-up of new skin cells. You look great when you're tanned and twenty, but sort of saggy and leathery when you have tanned for 70 years and skin cells no longer regenerate.

The high consumption of calcium in the form of supplements and dairy foods has been the game plan in American medicine for maintaining strong bones and preventing osteoporosis.

But excessive consumption of calcium overworks osteoblasts, and we only have so many that last only so long.

The blood calcium must remain at a constant level in order for the body to function properly. So deposits and withdrawals from the bones are made by osteoblasts (cells that store calcium and build bone matrix) and osteoclasts (cells that remove calcium from the bones and send it into the blood stream, or dispose of it in the urine). Sending lots of calcium into the body causes the excess to be stored in the bones.

Countries with high calcium diets have young people with very strong bones and old people with very weak bones. Osteoblasts are scurrying like rabbits to carry the excess calcium into the bones in people who supplement calcium and eat lots of dairy foods.

Osteoblasts lay down a matrix that will hold the calcium and make strong bones.

We all have only so many regenerative cells in our bodies. Finally for all of us, death is the result of losing all of our regenerative capabilities. If we overwork osteoblasts by sending excessive amounts of calcium into the body, the osteoblasts become like the rabbit. They are sprinting to an early death, making strong bones in youth, and weak bones in middle age and in the elderly as osteoblasts wear out.

Bones are living tissue that remodel to stress. When stress is applied to bones by walking and lifting and being active, the body reacts by osteoblastic activity and the laying down of strong bone material.

Sedentary people apply less stress to the bones and are susceptible to osteoporosis. The densest bone is the body is the heel bone because it strikes the earth every time you take a step. When American astronauts first went into space for weeks at a time, they experienced heel pain when they stepped off the space capsule after weeks of floating in space. With no heel striking, the body mobilized calcium away from the heels because it was not needed. This happened in a matter of weeks.

It is not the high consumption of calcium rich foods and the supplementing of calcium that lead to strong bones. We have tried that for many years. American women have been advised to eat lots of dairy foods, supplement calcium, exercise regularly, and take hormone replacement therapy.

Premarin was sold to post-menopausal women for 40 years because they were told it was necessary to prevent breast cancer, heart disease, and osteoporosis. When studies were finally conducted, it was discovered that women using premarin had a *higher* incidence of breast cancer, heart disease, and osteoporosis.

Americans consume more calcium and dairy foods than any country in the world, yet American women have the highest incidence of osteoporosis in the world. Chinese women do not get osteoporosis, yet they do not consume dairy foods. (have you ever seen any milk or cheese in Chinese restaurants?)

The main dietary cause of osteoporosis is too much protein in the diet. The American dinner plate consists of a few ounces of vegetables, maybe some beans or potatoes, and several ounces of some meat.

A Chinese meal consists of that same portion of meat, all chopped up, and mixed with rice and vegetables, enough to serve six or seven people. Less protein.

Many Americans worry about not getting enough protein when they should be concerned about getting too much protein. A high protein diet, and phosphates in carbonated beverages, deplete the body of calcium. It's not that we don't get enough calcium. We don't absorb enough with a diet of too much protein and sodas.

Dr. Frank Oski and Dr. John McDougall point out that milk, although rich in calcium, also contains a lot of phosphate, is high in protein, and actually provides a net calcium loss.

It is not necessary to consume dairy foods to prevent osteoporosis. Cows have strong bones, and they are herbivores. They don't drink milk after they are weaned.

Dairy foods cause most chronic pain.

Vegetarian people all over the earth have strong bones without consuming dairy foods, and they don't supplement calcium.

The use of Fosamax and Evitra to inhibit osteoclast activity is a huge mistake. Osteoclasts are essential for mobilizing calcium which is needed all over the body.

The most effective way to keep bones as strong as you can for as long as you can is to:

1. Decrease your intake of protein foods (meat, eggs, dairy foods)
2. Drink no carbonated beverages
3. Walk regularly (applying stress to the skeleton).

Osteoporosis and high cholesterol are preventable.

We are sold the notion that expensive, harmful drugs are the only answer to these problems.

The solution is diet and exercise and the specific changes outlined in Part One of this book.

4. Gluten Intolerance and Pain

Gluten is the main protein found in wheat. It is also found in barley and rye and semolina in pasta.

Gluten is an allergen that causes inflammatory problems in some people who are sensitive to it.

More people are allergic to dairy foods. Dairy food sensitivity (allergy to casein) makes sense because cow's milk is the perfect nutrient for baby cows, not humans.

But the logic of gluten intolerance is not apparent at first.

Many people have various inflammatory reactions to dairy foods. The same inflammatory reactions, in fact any inflammatory reaction, can be caused by gluten when an individual has inherited, or developed the trait of gluten intolerance.

Known also as celiac disease, gluten intolerance has been around for thousands of years. But it still seems to defy logic that people can react poorly to wheat, the staff of life.

Al Gore mentions a possible explanation is his 1986 book, *Earth in the Balance.* The original seeds of the various plant foods of the world, the plants that support human life on our planet, originated in specific "centers of diversity." The night-shade vegetables, which include tomatoes and potatoes and peppers, originated in the new world in Central and South America.

Those foods did not make their way to Europe until the 1500's when Spanish explorers discovered the people of North, Central, and South America. Aztecs, Mayas, and Incans were building complex, advanced, and technical societies while Europe muddled through the Dark Ages.

After nightshade vegetables made their way into the diets of Europeans, potatoes in the north, tomatoes in the south, the Renaissance movement began. Some people, like Anemarie Colbin have written about that phenomenon and suspect that the alkaloids in night shade vegetables, which stimulate abstract thought, could have been responsible.

The original wheat plants and seeds originated in Mesopotamia (the Middle East). The wild strains of wheat that originated there do not resemble the domesticated wheat that has changed genetically over time through natural selection and breeding by farmers who were seeking the hardiest, most productive plants.

While the genetics of the wheat plants changed over time, the genetics of humans changed much more slowly, and some people could not adapt to the new strains of wheat. They had digestive problems, and now we are learning, neurological and musculoskeletal symptoms and skin reactions.

You may have noticed that gluten intolerance is mentioned more often now in health and even medical literature. Many grocery stores now stock gluten free products, and some even have gluten free aisles and sections. All health food stores carry gluten free products.

Gluten intolerance is four times more prevalent now than it was in the 1950's. This is due to an increased awareness by a better educated public, but also due to more radical changes in wheat itself.

Norman Borlaug saved billions of lives by creating a new strain of wheat that was hardier, more productive, and more resistant to pests. He earned the Nobel Prize for his efforts.

Norman Borlaug recognized the desperation of the situation in the world in the 1940's when millions of people were starving. Waiting for the different strains to be produced through breeding seemed too time consuming as the world population grew and starvation of millions of people was imminent. So Borlaug used x-rays and gamma rays to mutate wheat seeds to increase the number of mutations and speed up the process of finding a better seed and plant. Most mutations are bad, but rare ones are good.

He found one that produced hardy plants that produced more wheat and were resistant to pests. Wheat production in the world was massively increased and lives were saved.

Because of the radical change in the wheat plant, today there are many more people who cannot tolerate the new breed. While most people are nourished by wheat, a few are sensitive to the protein.

The same is true of medications, powerful chemicals that seem to help most people, but cause serious side effects in others. Penicillin was a miracle antibiotic for millions of people who were dieing of pneumonia and other infectious diseases when it was developed in 1928 by Alexander Fleming.

But some people are sensitive to penicillin and could die from just one small dose.

People who suffer with chronic pain are more likely to suffer with gluten intolerance than people who have no symptoms. So in the thorough management of chronic pain, gluten intolerance must be an important consideration in the treatment program.

When you suffer with chronic pain, and you know how unsuccessful conventional medicine has been on your behalf, there is no time to mess around and *consider* other options.

It is time to eliminate all allergens and toxins that could possibly be contributing to your pain or health problems. There are other allergens that, in rare cases, cause inflammatory reactions like chronic pain. Pain can also be caused by night shade vegetables, corn, soy, or sugar.

Gluten and casein are the most common allergens that contribute to health problems like chronic pain, headaches, skin problems, fibromyalgia, lupus, mental problems, digestive upset, female problems like infertility and endometriosis, and on and on.

Any health problem must be addressed with the elimination of food allergens.

Gluten and casein must be eliminated in all cases of chronic pain.

5. Monosodium Glutamate is a Nerve Toxin
(and so is Aspartame)

Monosodium glutamate (MSG) is a flavor enhancer found in processed foods, and is naturally occurring in seaweed. The Japanese have used seaweed as a seasoning for thousands of years.

Kikunae Ikeda was able to isolate the chemical component of seaweed that was responsible for the strong seasoning sensation. He found that the flavor was due to the amino acid **glutamic acid** combined with sodium to produce a salt: monosodium glutamate. He received a patent for it in 1909.

By 1933 the Japanese were producing 10 million pounds of MSG each year. They tried to sell it to American food producers, but were unsuccessful until 1948. When American food manufacturers were shown that MSG eliminated the tin can taste of canned foods, they jumped on board.

By the 1950's, many American housewives were using Accent™ on every dish. Pure spices like salt, pepper, fennel, oregano, dill, etc. are natural substances. Spices that are mixtures, like Taco seasoning, Italian seasoning, and Lemon-pepper list ingredients on the label that may include MSG or a form of it. Accent™ lists one ingredient because Accent™ is pure MSG.

In 1957 food manufacturers became more proficient at producing MSG by using a fermentation process in which bacteria were used to produce MSG. The cheaper product led to wider use.

The use of MSG has grown astronomically in this country since then. Americans now consume 80 million pounds of MSG annually.

MSG is found in many processed foods and in restaurants. Steps 4 and 7 in the first part of this book are essential for the elimination of chronic pain. Avoiding processed foods and restaurant food is mainly because of MSG.

The sensation of taste involves nerve tissue in the nose, mouth, and the brain. The taste buds are embedded with nerve fibers that carry the sensation of taste to the brain. They detect sweet, sour, beefy, salty, bitter, and other taste sensations, and a nerve impulse is sent to the brain where it is interpreted.

Once MSG has stimulated the taste buds, it goes through the digestive tract and is eventually absorbed into the blood stream where it makes its way to all of the cells in the body. Animal studies have shown that MSG is a powerful nerve toxin, causing nerves to swell immediately upon contact. Widespread damage occurs in the dendrites, the filaments that transfer electrical impulses to other nerves and the brain.

When the damage occurs throughout the brain and central nervous system, the effects can cause virtually any neurological disorder, from severe pain anywhere in the body, digestive upset, loss of memory, inability to concentrate, mood changes, and dementia.

Consider all of the neurological disorders with no known causes that can't be explained: migraines, schizophrenia, multiple sclerosis, Parkinson's disease, Alzheimer's, carpal tunnel syndrome, Lou Gehrig's disease, Huntington's chorea, etc. The list is long, and none of these disease processes has been adequately explained by modern medicine.

Conventional medicine has yet to consider the diet for anything beyond obesity, or very clumsily, for diabetes.

The premise of this book is that disease processes are caused by allergens and toxins that cause inflammatory reactions that lead to a series of chemical events that cause misery and eventual death.

When conventional medicine doesn't work (and it doesn't for chronic pain and these diseases of minor and severe neuro-funk), it's way past time for the doctors to ask "what do you eat?" And maybe the medication this patient is using might be responsible for the symptoms that are clearly listed as possible side effects.

But no.

MSG has no taste of its own, maybe slightly salty or bitter. But MSG acts as a nerve stimulator by irritating the nerve fibers in the taste buds, thus enhancing the taste signal sent to the brain. The brain receives a much stronger signal and enhances the flavor of almost any food.

The sweet taste sensation does not appear to be enhanced by MSG, so most dessert foods and fruit drinks do not contain MSG. The sweet taste buds are stimulated by sugar foods and artificially by aspartame.

Aspartame is very similar in chemical structure to MSG. Aspartame stimulates the sweet taste buds, even though it contains no sugar, and no calories. The belief that consuming this nerve toxin is great for losing weight is false. There are so many dangers to consuming any nerve toxin that using aspartame or MSG is a risk that far outweighs the imagined benefit.

The history of aspartame approval by the FDA is one of corruption and possible bribery. Aspartame has spawned a billion dollar industry that is harming people more than it benefits anyone's health. Researchers in the 1970's found that aspartame produced brain tumors in rats, but the FDA somehow approved it for public use. New research is showing problems with diet foods containing aspartame.

Most chewing gum, diet sodas, low-sugar foods, and no-sugar foods contain aspartame and must be avoided to end chronic pain and any neurological disorder.

While aspartame is a nerve toxin, MSG is much more common at causing chronic pain.

Public awareness of MSG has grown, but not nearly enough. Many people have told me they thought MSG had been banned. Not true by a long shot. (Check out "MSG is Everywhere" by me). Because more and more people are becoming aware, manufacturers are hiding the fact that MSG is in their products.

The following products used in processed foods contain MSG:

Monosodium glutamate
Hydrolyzed protein (any kind)
Calcium caseinate
Sodium caseinate
Yeast extract
Autolyzed yeast
Gelatin
Textured Vegetable Protein (TVP found in processed vegetarian foods)
Protein isolate (in most protein shakes)

The notion that heavily processed protein supplements are healthy and necessary for body-building is a myth.

Frank V. was a very healthy 42 year old who cycled and ran every day. He competed in cycling and running and triathalon events. He limped with severe right sciatic pain. Therapy and the elimination of dairy foods and MSG did not solve his problem. It was the elimination of his protein shake that contained protein isolate as the second ingredient that made his chronic sciatic pain go away.

MSG **may** be in the following:

> Natural flavors
> Natural flavorings
> Spices
> Carrageenan
> Pectin
> Seasonings

Ingredient labels are supposed to inform consumers, but they very often mislead consumers. Because of this, it is best to just avoid processed foods and restaurants. (See page 167)

MSG is found mainly in packaged, processed foods, snack foods, TV Dinners, processed meats, canned and dry soup, salad dressing, many spices, and in restaurant food. It is used in some vitamins and medication where it is listed as hydrolyzed protein.

Packaged Foods

Almost all frozen TV Dinners contain MSG, even the supposedly healthy brands like Jenny Craig™, Weight Watchers™, Healthy Choice™, and Nutrisystems™. Foods that are frozen for long periods of time lose much of their flavor. MSG is used to enhance the dulled flavor of these frozen entrees.

Any food that is advertised as spicier, zestier, or having a fuller flavor, or a bolder flavor, likely contains MSG. Pure rice, whether it is white or brown, is a pure food. White rice has been polished and stripped of some nutrients, but no artificial chemicals have been added.

Spicier rices, like Rice-a-Roni™ and rice pilaf in restaurants are flavored with MSG. Uncle Ben's™ flavored rice also contains MSG.

Almost any packaged food used to enhance a meal contains MSG. Stove Top Stuffing Mix™, Hamburger Helper™, Shake and Bake™, etc. almost always contain MSG. Any sauce packet, or seasoning packet or mix is very likely to contain MSG.

Processed Meat

The pure meats at the butcher counter are not usually chemically treated with a flavor enhancer. Fresh hamburger, steaks, pork, lamb, chicken, turkey, fish, etc. are usually safe, as far as MSG is concerned. However, some of the cheap hamburger meat in opaque wrapping contains MSG.

Most ground turkey contains MSG and is listed as Natural Flavors or hydrolyzed protein. Frozen turkey is injected with hydrolyzed protein.

While there are no labels on the meat at the butcher counter, all of the meats at the deli counter are labeled because they are chemically treated with MSG and many other chemicals that are suspected carcinogens, like nitrates and nitrites. Deli meats like salami, boloney, pastrami, ham, turkey ham, chorizo, kobassa, bacon, sausage, and canned meat spreads usually contain MSG.

Most bacon has a very small dose of MSG, and some bacon has no MSG. Almost all sausage contains MSG, and usually a high dose.

Lunch meats often contain MSG. The cheaper brands are likely to use more MSG than the expensive brands. Patients who react to MSG have more problems with Carl Buddig™, generic, and store brands than they do with Oscar Mayer™ and Louis Rich™.

104

Most canned tuna contains MSG, listed as hydrolyzed protein, hydrolyzed casein, but usually listed as vegetable broth. Currently there are several brands that don't contain MSG. Low sodium tuna contains only tuna and water. You may find it on the diet aisle with the Slim Fast™ and diet foods.

Bumble Bee makes a low sodium variety and a solid white albacore that contains no MSG. Both cans are gold, as of this writing, but they change all the time. Pyrophosphate is a preservative in some of these products, but is not MSG.

Lots of restaurants use some MSG and some restaurants use lots of MSG. Chinese food, Thai food, and Japanese food usually use large doses of MSG. Sushi is wrapped in seaweed and contains MSG. Breaded foods usually contain MSG in the breading.

Kentucky Fried Chicken™ uses lots of MSG in its breading. Pulling off the skin does not eliminate the MSG (we know, we've tried it). Chicken Nuggets, breaded seafood, country fried steak, and fish sticks are breaded and usually contain MSG.

Sauces used to add flavor to meats and other dishes, like Teriaki sauce, soy sauce, au jus on prime rib, and BBQ sauce usually contain MSG. The best tasting BBQ sauces use the most MSG. Patients who react to MSG react more severely to Masterpiece™, Bull's Eye™, and Chris n' Pits™ brands of BBQ sauce.

Patients with MSG sensitivity also react very severely when they eat at In n' Out Burger™. MSG is in the sauce on their burgers.

Most soups and broths contain MSG. Swanson's™ makes a broth that claims "No MSG added." It contains yeast extract, which contains MSG.

Panda Express™ has a sign at the front of their line that reads, "We add no MSG." Patients who are sensitive to MSG react after eating at Panda Express™. They don't add it because many of their foods already contain MSG.

Flavored snack foods contain MSG. Regular potato chips and corn chips contain no MSG. But almost all flavored chips, like sour cream and onion, barbeque chips, *red hot cheetos™*, *cheetos™*, *gold fish™*, and any other flavor available usually contains MSG. (see page 182)

Many manufacturers are now offering foods that actually don't contain any MSG. Most Lawry's™ spices contain no MSG.

Lawry's Seasoning Salt™ is a versatile spice that contains no MSG.

Mrs. Dash™ spices contain no MSG.

Many restaurants claim they don't use MSG, but I have seen MSG sensitive patients react at some of them. Many restaurants are not aware that some of the foods they buy contain MSG.

The Olive Garden Restaurant™ makes the claim of no MSG in their soups, and so far I have seen no reactions. So currently, I take them at their word.

But things change.

Campbell's™ used to make a soup called Healthy Request™ that actually had no MSG. The can had a blue stripe around the can with the words "Healthy Request" on the stripe. (see page 178). A few years back they changed the color of the stripe to green, still labeled it as Healthy Request, but added MSG back into the soup. (See page 177)

Currently, I know of no canned or packaged soup that does not contain MSG. Swanson's™ makes a broth that's labeled "No MSG Added" but is contains MSG in yeast extract (see page 69).

MSG reactions are dose dependant. MSG is a toxin, and all toxins cause reactions, and all toxins are dose dependant. For example, alcohol is toxic to the nervous system: A little will make you tipsy, more will make you say things you'll regret, even more and you pass out, and if you drink way too much you will die. Some college kids failed to graduate because of it.

MSG is a toxin that will cause a reaction in any human being if he dose is high enough. It has been assumed that most people will not react to a small dose of MSG. But many people are suffering with problems that are due to MSG and they don't even know it.

A high dose of MSG can come from a food with a lot of MSG, like Chinese food, restaurant soup, Top Ramen™, KFC™, sausage, in one dose. You might feel sick afterward, get a headache, or fell depressed. A large dose can also be applied a little at a time in several meals for several days in a row. The first meal may not cause a noticeable reaction, but a subsequent meal or meals may be enough to reach a dose that causes a noticeable and unpleasant reaction.

People who eat out a lot are susceptible to long term exposure to small or big, but regular doses of MSG that will cause neurological damage and subsequent health problems, including chronic pain.

Taco Bell™ meat contains autolyzed yeast extract, a source of MSG. It also contains cocoa powder, and will cause reactions in people who are sensitive to chocolate, the most powerful cause of pain.

MSG Reactions

Chest Pain

The most common reaction to MSG looks like a heart attack. Shortly after the meal, and even as late as 24 hours after a meal with MSG, the patient will experience chest pain, palpitations and shortness of breath. They may get nauseous and throw up.

By the time these patients have been rushed to the hospital and checked, they feel better and are diagnosed with panic disorder.

Panic Attacks

Most panic attacks are caused by MSG. Most people realize that the circumstances preceding the event do not call for panic. The reaction is purely chemical.

Other allergens and toxins can cause this neurological reaction but most panic and anxiety attacks are caused by MSG.

Mood Changes

Unexplained or poorly justified depression, or outbursts of anger are very often caused by MSG

Headaches

All headaches are chemical reactions. After dairy foods (casein) and chocolate, MSG is the most common cause of headaches.

Most headaches are caused by:

> Casein
> Chocolate
> MSG
> Aspartame
> Medication
> Gluten

> ...in that order.

Neck, shoulder, and arm pain:
These symptoms, including numbness in the extremities are common reactions to MSG.

> When MSG is the cause of this form of neuro-funk, symptoms are on the left 75% of the time.

Sciatic Pain

Hand Swelling and Numbness

Fibromyalgia Symptoms

Nightmares

Mysterious Bruises (usually about the size of a dime)

Fullness in the throat

You may not have noticeable symptoms to MSG (except maybe you just don't feel "quite right") unless the dose is very high. But MSG is a toxin that may be causing problems that you won't notice until it is too late.

Many reactions are sub-clinical: mood changes, inability to concentrate or remember things, irritability, depression, negativity, chronic fatigue, and on and on.

MSG is a nerve toxin that destroys nerve tissue, and while you are young and have a plethora of healthy nervous tissue, you can binge drink and survive MSG with no noticeable reaction until that plethora of healthy nerves is whittled down as you age, until fine motor movements are compromised, memory fades, vision gets weak, headaches are more frequent. Then one day your wife notices the tremors, the head and hand shaking.

Many people later discover symptoms they never knew they had until they quit using MSG. People who give it up are often more energetic, nicer human beings. Their reading comprehension improves, their memory improves, and they become more optimistic. They see better.

We all know that many crimes and moral decadence are caused by drugs and alcohol.

Prison diets consist mainly of caffeine and Top Ramen™, which is loaded with MSG. These people already have behavior problems.

How can we explain the poor performance of our kids in school? Their behavior? (see page 182 for one of the most common snacks at school)

Of course there are lots of reasons, but just check out what kids are eating at school. They have lots of choices and all of them are bad.

Baby food manufacturers agreed to eliminate MSG from baby food in 1968. But most school lunch programs contain MSG. And when kids bypass the lunch counter for those red hot cheetos™, they are getting a huge dose of neurotoxin.

MSG is in our school lunches. MSG is widely used in our prisons where inmates consume and trade Top Ramen™ in huge quantities.

For God's sake, MSG is used in hospital food where it is fed to people who are already sick.

Restaurants, grocery stores, and health food stores are loaded with MSG.

MSG is everywhere.

In order to eliminate chronic pain, MSG must be eliminated.

6. Headaches

Headaches have two causes:

> 1. **Exposure** to some substance, an allergen or a toxin.

> 2. **Withdrawal** from some substance, allergen or toxin.

Casein in dairy foods is the most common cause of chronic headaches.

Chocolate is included in dairy foods, even chocolate that contains no milk.

Chocolate is a very common cause of headaches.

Monosodium glutamate is the next most common cause of headaches.

Aspartame in gums and diet foods can cause headaches.

Casein in dairy foods, caseinate in non-dairy foods, chocolate, MSG, and aspartame cause 90% of all headaches.

The next most common cause of chronic pain is medication.

Many drugs list headaches as a side effect (see page 132).

Hangovers are sometimes withdrawal from alcohol, and sometimes they are due to exposure and poisoning to too much of the toxic substance: alcohol.

After that, exposure to gluten (wheat), corn (and corn additives like corn meal, corn syrup, etc.), soy, night shade vegetables (tomatoes, potatoes, egg plant, red and green bell peppers) can cause headaches, but rarely.

But "rarely" doesn't matter if these allergens cause headaches for you.

Chocolate is the most powerful cause of pain.

Inhaled substances like cigarette smoke, perfumes, carbon monoxide, formaldehyde, and other substances can cause headaches.

Caffeine can cause headaches both coming and going:

>**Exposure** to caffeine can cause headaches.

>**Withdrawal** from caffeine can cause headaches.

Regular coffee (or soda) drinkers can have constant headaches both from exposure to and withdrawal from caffeine.

People who drink coffee regularly have probably experienced the caffeine withdrawal headache after quitting coffee, or missing their daily dose.

Withdrawal from any allergen or toxin can cause headaches.

Quitting dairy foods, chocolate, MSG, aspartame, other allergens, and drugs can cause headaches.

Withdrawal usually lasts 3-4 days, up to a week, and sometimes a little longer.

Classifying headaches (cluster, migraine, stress, etc.) is pointless. CT scans and MRI's and x-rays are almost always negative.

If a dreaded tumor is apparent in these imaging studies, it is the result (another symptom) of chronic exposure to the allergen or toxin that is causing the headaches.

Headaches can be caused by trauma, but not chronic headaches.

To eliminate headaches, refer to part one and follow those instructions.

7. Autoimmune Diseases Are Not

Autoimmune diseases are included in this book because they are diseases of hopelessness, they are painful, and they're chronic. The text books are full of them, and they are described in great detail, but have no solution beyond being classified as chronic.

It is assumed that these diseases are caused by some glitch in the immune system where self-tissue is attacked for some unknown reason. That is speculation, and if you read the text books describing these autoimmune diseases, you will see lots of "could be," "maybe," "probably," "unknown," "elusive," and "it is thought that, although...."

Autoimmune diseases are defined as reactions of the immune system against the body's own tissue. Autoimmune diseases, and the whole process itself, are poorly understood. Consequently, treatment is ineffective and involves only drugs, immunosuppressors, that suppress the entire immune response. This compromises the ability to fight infection and other allergens, and interferes with healing in general.

Powerful drugs like prednisone and enbrel cause serious side effects, including death.

The diet is never considered as a solution for autoimmune diseases.

Autoimmune diseases are not reactions against the self, but reactions against allergens that have been ingested or inhaled or absorbed through the skin. These reactions occur in people who are genetically pre-disposed to the disease.

Consider this from Robbins Textbook, Pathologic Basis of Disease:

115

Rheumatoid arthritis (RA)

Pathogenesis. It is believed that RA is an autoimmune disease triggered by exposure of a genetically susceptible host to an unknown arthritogenic antigen. (Robbins 1306)

The autoimmune reaction in RA consists of activated CD4+ T cells, and probably B lymphocytes, as well. The target antigens of these lymphocytes, and how they are initially activated, are still unknown. (Robbins 1307)

Although the cause of RA remains unknown, autoimmunity plays a pivotal role in its chronicity and progression. (Robbins 1305)

Examples of organ specific autoimmunity are type I diabetes mellitus, in which the autoreactive T cells and antibodies are specific for beta cells of the pancreatic islets, and multiple sclerosis, in which autoreactive T cells react against the central nervous system myelin. (Robbins 223)

An example of systemic autoimmune disease is SLE (systemic lupus erythematosis. (Robbins 223)

Humans live in an environment teeming with substances capable of producing immunologic responses. Contact with antigen leads not only to induction of a protective immune response, but also to reactions that can be damaging to tissues.

Exogenous antigens occur in dust, pollens, foods, drugs, microbiologic agents, chemicals, and many blood products used in chemical practice. (Robbins 205)

...the hypersensitivity reaction results from the binding of antibodies to normal or altered cell-surface antigens. (Robbins 210)

To summarize **Robbins**: Rheumatoid arthritis (and other autoimmune diseases) is an inflammatory reaction mediated by an immune response.

The immune system reacts to antigens (allergens) that enter the body and set off the inflammatory response.

So called autoimmune reactions are immune reactions to antigens (allergens) that have been bound to cells of the host, like in the joints, the airways, the nervous system, anywhere.

Rheumatoid arthritis (and many other diseases called autoimmune) are reactions to antigens that have been ingested.

The "unknown" antigens are dietary allergens.

These diseases are due to the diet, the one taboo area to medical doctors.

Robbins Pathological Basis of Disease, Seventh Edition copyright 2005, Elsevier, Inc.

Diabetes

Many diabetics know that, in their case, eliminating sugar and simple carbohydrates from the diet does not lower blood sugar. Medication or insulin is the only alternative in modern medicine.

But Dr. William Philpot discovered that sugar levels can be affected by foods containing little or no carbohydrate. He was able to affect sugar levels in one patient with cream cheese, a dairy food that is only 2% carbohydrate.

He concluded: *"The assumption that these disordered carbohydrate reactions will be in response to carbohydrate*

117

only is not valid. Testing reveals that they occur to any type of food and that the central cause is that of being allergic to or in a specific way to a specified food, whether fat, protein, or carbohydrate." (Foreman, 190)

Multiple Sclerosis

In the textbook by Robbins: *Multiple sclerosis is an autoimmune demyelinating disorder characterized by distinct episodes of neurologic deficits...*

Pathogenesis: The lesions of MS are caused by a cellular immune response that is inappropriately directed against the components of the myelin sheath. The likelihood of developing this autoimmune process is influenced by genetic and environmental factors. (Robbins 1383)

The available evidence indicates that the disease is initiated by CD4+ T cells that react against self myelin antigens. (Robbins 1383)

Little sclerotic (hard) plaques are the result of the inflammatory reaction. These hard spots along the nerve interfere with nerve conduction and contribute to the neuro-funk of the disease: trouble walking, swallowing, problems with coordination, etc.

These sclerotic plaques cannot be healed. However, the immune reaction is not to the self, but to an ingested allergen that **can** be avoided. When the allergen is avoided, the disease will stop progressing.

When we talk about neuro-funk, we have to discuss Parkinson's Disease (PD).

Parkinsonism is a clinical disorder characterized by diminished facial expression, stooped posture, slowness of

118

oluntary movement, *festinating gait (progressively shortened, ccelerated steps), rigidity, and a pill rolling tremor* (of the ands). (Robbins 1391) (see Muhammed Ali)

hese symptoms are caused by degeneration of a part of the rain called the substantia nigra. No one is sure what causes iis degeneration, but ...*evidence has also suggested that esticide exposure may increase the risk of PD, while caffeine nd nicotine may be protective.* (Robbins 1392)

Jothing definitive is suggested here, but degeneration is the esult of ongoing inflammation, and inflammation is caused by llergens and toxins. Researchers have noticed that this disease s affected by environmental and dietary factors.

₋ots of other supposedly autoimmune diseases, like myas- henia gravis, Graves disease, ulcerative colitis, systemic lupus rythematosis, scleroderma, and others, are immune reactions, ut **not to the self**.

'soriasis is another chronic disease initiated by an immune esponse. It needs no description if you have it, but it is lescribed as *a chronic inflammatory dermatosis* (skin ondition). (Robbins 1256)

²athogenesis. Psoriasis is a T-cell mediated disease..." Robbins 1257)

Robbins concludes: *As with many other autoimmune diseases, he antigen that triggers the immune response remains elusive.* Robbins 1257)

The cause of these diseases is elusive because conventional nedicine:

Considers drugs as the only tool.

Does not consider the diet.

These autoimmune diseases are considered mysteriou reactions against the self.

The allergens are elusive because they are usually dietar factors.

Dave came into my office in May of 1992. He complained o right knee swelling and chronic headaches. I had him take of his pants and this is what I saw:

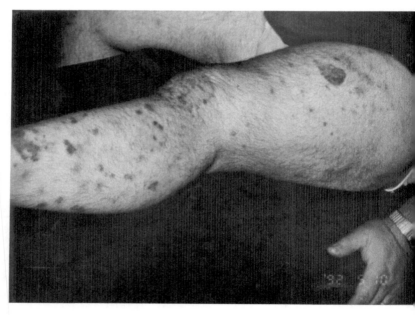

Dave had psoriasis, an incurable disease, an autoimmune disease. Note the date, May 10, 1992.

In color, those lesions are bright red with inflammation.

To eliminate his headaches, I instructed Dave to eliminate all dairy foods.

We started a course of chiropractic care and physical therapy.

This picture was taken one month later on 6/15/92.

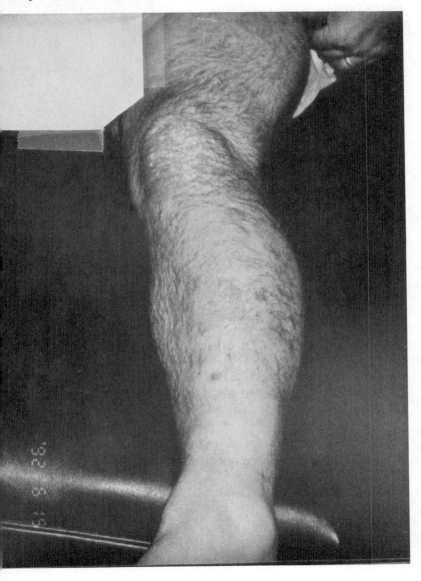

The red lesions have faded and are starting to dry up.

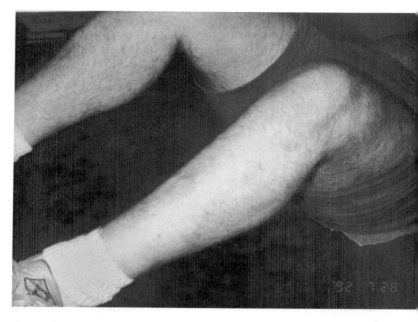

On July 7, 1992, less than 90 days after eliminating dairy foods, there is no inflammation.

This case of psoriasis was allergy: not to his own tissue, but to the casein in dairy foods.

Doctors never considered his diet, just steroid creams and the advice to "learn to live with it."

Diet should be considered in all cases of "autoimmunity." After all, diet changes are not dangerous.

Prednisone is dangerous, especially when taken chronically for chronic conditions.

8.   The Rules of Diet Manipulation

Food allergens:

The most common food allergens causing pain are:

> Casein
> Chocolate
> Gluten

Other possible allergens causing pain are:

> Soy
> Corn
> Cane Sugar

> Night Shade Vegetables:
>
> > Tomatoes
> > Potatoes
> > Red and Green Bell Peppers

The most common toxins causing chronic pain are:

> Monosodium glutamate (MSG)
> Aspartame
> Medication

Toxic reactions are dose dependant.

Allergic reactions are *not* dose dependant.

All of the allergen must be avoided 100%.

It's not how much, but how often you consume an allergen:

> A little milk on your cereal several times a week,
> cream in your coffee every day,
> cheese several times a week,
> only a little bit of chocolate.....

These small doses are enough to keep you in chronic pain.

Each dose (a splash of milk, a slice of cheese, etc.) will cause an inflammatory reaction that will last for 3, 4, or 5 days, up to a week.

So exposure to an allergen *only* twice a week can cause chronic, ongoing symptoms.

Reaction time to an allergen can be from instantly, up to 48 hours.

The most common reaction time is 2 to 12 hours.

A reaction to supper may occur in the middle of the night, or shortly after rising.

A chocolate dessert in the evening may cause severe lower back pain when you are in the shower the next morning.....

....or a headache that comes on after you get to work.

Reaction time and recovery time are usually not instantaneous.

It's like starting and stopping a locomotive...it takes a while.

9. What to expect in 90 days:

Once you completely eliminate the allergens and toxins that are causing your pain, the following events occur:

Days 1-7: Withdrawal:

> You may feel worse.
> Headaches and flu and cold symptoms are common.
> Your symptoms may not change at all.

The first seven days are the most difficult.

You may have ups and downs in the first week.

You may not get better at all in the first week, and you may feel worse.

Days 7 - 30: Symptoms improve, and sensitivity increases.

> Symptoms will improve slowly or rapidly during this time.

> Any exposure to the trigger during this time, and in the first 60 days, will cause a more severe reaction.

Days 30-90: Symptoms improve, other symptoms improve, and sensitivity decreases (in most cases) during this time.

> Symptoms will continue to improve.

> You will notice other improvements:

>> Skin
>> Energy level
>> Digestion
>> Sinuses clearing
>> Moods

>>> And more.

Withdrawal

Many people will experience withdrawal symptoms in the first week or so of avoidance.

The mechanism of food causing pain is an action of the immune system, called allergy by many. These reactions are more accurately called **allergy-addiction.**

When an allergen or toxin is suddenly eliminated, the body will often go into withdrawal.

Quitting coffee (caffeine) is an example. If you drink coffee regularly, then one day quit, or don't get your coffee, you are likely to get a headache.

This is caffeine withdrawal.

This could happen if you quit any allergen or toxin: heroin, cigarettes, alcohol (DT's), medications, casein, gluten, etc.

Common withdrawal symptoms are:

> Headache
> Overall soreness
> A worsening of pain
> Lousy feeling
> Flu and cold symptoms
> Tiredness

Typical withdrawal is on day 3 and day 4.

But withdrawal could last up to two weeks.

Chronic pain will be gone in 90 days.

Total healing will continue even after 90 days.

Craving

Many people think craving something is a sign that you need that something. That is not true.

The body of a heroin addict does not *need* heroin. Likewise with cigarettes, alcohol, etc.

When an allergen or toxin is discontinued, withdrawal symptoms begin. The body knows that there are only two ways out of withdrawal:

1. Riding out the miserable symptoms for a few days or weeks.

2. Taking a dose of the allergen or toxin.

The withdrawal symptoms can be stopped by taking a small dose of the allergen or toxin.

The body doesn't really want to experience withdrawal, so you get a craving for the dose that will end the misery. This is called a **neutralizing dose** "(hair of the dog)".

Increased sensitivity (7 - 30 or 60 days)

During the first few weeks and perhaps months, any exposure to a trigger will cause a more severe reaction. When you suffer with chronic pain caused by regular exposure to the allergen or toxin, your body makes an attempt to adapt.

But once exposure stops and healing begins, sensitivity will increase. When casein causes chronic pain, a glass of milk or a piece of cheese or some ranch dressing during the first few weeks or months will cause more severe pain, and maybe even a different reaction.

Regular coffee drinkers usually don't get wired from th coffee. They can drink a cup and go to bed and go right t sleep if they want.

But if they quit coffee, they will get a withdrawal headache fo a while, maybe feel like they can't get going for a while, the they recover. Energy returns even without their caffeine fix.

But one cup of coffee after several weeks of abstinence wil hype them up and give them the jitters.

The increased sensitivity is usually temporary and is followed by a decrease in sensitivity.

Decreased sensitivity (90 days and beyond)

Most people will experience a decreased sensitivity the longe they avoid the allergens and toxins that caused their pain.

After 90 days of avoidance, they may be able to tolerate small doses of the allergen on rare occasions.

If your pain improved after avoiding an allergen, it is best to avoid it altogether, forever.

But most people will be able to have some of the allergen once a week, but no more than once a week....twice a month is safer.

Some people (20%) with a sensitivity will have a noticeable reaction each and every time they eat the allergen....forever.

The Phenomenon of Changing Symptoms

After 90 days of elimination, future exposure will often cause a different reaction.

For example, if you had headaches that were solved by eliminating casein in dairy foods, future exposure after 90 days could cause a different symptom, perhaps lower back pain, or elbow pain.

The allergen has no loyalty to symptoms, just to elevated inflammation.

Once healing has taken place (90 days) the inflamed tissue is stronger, and the allergen could cause inflammation that would spill over at another, now weaker area.

10. Drugs Cause Side Effects (including pain)

Is it possible for a pharmaceutical concoction, that wa designed for one effect, to actually cause another reaction perhaps a side effect?

Pharmaceutical labs have been buzzing for years, torturing rat and other innocent beasts. Researchers found that on substance injected into rats caused them to become lethargic lose interest in mating, become thirsty, gain body weight, anc lower their blood pressure. A light bulb went on when the consulted the list of 161 risk factors for heart disease:

> "Hey, we can lower blood pressure!"

Today, 25 million Americans are taking blood pressure medi cation. The use of lisinopril, atenelol, hydrochlorothiazide diovan, tenormin, and many other drugs that lower blooc pressure have created another cottage industry: erectile dys function and the new drugs that are used to treat *that* disorder.

A recent commercial by a drug company that airs during prime time in this TV nation shows men who "just asked thei doctors" and found out what they didn't know: "I didn't know high blood pressure could cause erectile dysfunction?" Anothe perplexed male in the same commercial adds fuel to the fire with what he didn't know, "that diabetes could cause erectile dysfunction." Impotence is a clearly listed side effect of blood pressure medication in up to 42% of users.

It's not that one disease causes the other. The facts are that sick individuals may have all kinds of problems that are caused by their diets and lifestyles and medications.

The dark and doomed drug path that ensues after you consult your doctor, or just "ask your doctor" leads to many other

130

health problems and side effects that take a patient to an early, bloated, and miserable demise. Not a pretty picture.

This new book was written so I could include this chapter , a compilation of case studies of patients who had health problems that were caused by their diets and medications their doctors prescribed for them.

And this is especially a heads-up to medical professionals who may be beating their heads against a wall, and getting no results with physical medicine and their usual case management. Many chronic pain symptoms are merely side effects to medication, and if that is not addressed, the patient will not respond.

Big pharma keeps inventing drugs that are designed to fight the effects of the standard American diet and lifestyle.

Musculoskeletal symptoms, like back pain, neck pain, numbness and tingling in the extremities (paresthesias), and headaches do not respond well to conventional medicine.

The following drugs are the 15 most prescribed drugs:

Vicodin (for pain)
*Zocor (symvastatin) (for cholesterol)
*Lisinopril (blood pressure)
*Levothyroxine (thyroid)
*Azithromycin (antibiotic)
*Metformin (diabetes)
*Lipitor (cholesterol)
*Norvasc (blood pressure)
Amoxicillin (antibiotic)
Hydrochlorothiazide (blood pressure)
Prilosec (heartburn)
Xanax (depression)
Lasix (blood thinner)
*Metoprolol (blood pressure)
*Atenelol (blood pressure)

The ones with asterisks list **headaches** as a possible side effect. Many, many more drugs also list headaches as side effects.

Paresthesias are abnormal nerve sensations (sometimes called neuropathy), like numbness, pain, and tingling, usually in the extremities. Conventional medicine considers these symptoms as pinched nerves, requiring manipulation, surgery, or other drugs like neurontin.

The following drugs list **paresthesias** as a possible side effect:

Prozac	Lisinopril	Trazadone
Xanax	Buspar	Norvasc
Effexor	Diovan	Plavix
Flexeril	Motrin	Depo-provera
Crestor	Wellbutrin	
Procardia	Celexa	

After the common cold, **back pain** is the most common complaint that drives people to seek medical help. While there are many treatments for chronic back pain, most of them are temporary or ineffective.

The following list includes *some* of the drugs that list back pain as a possible side effect:

Zocor	Lipitor
Levitra	Flomax
Nexium	Cipro
Lexapro	Viagara
Effexor	Niacin
Progesterone	Zoloft
Estrace	Wellbutrin
Cialis	Excedrin
Topomax	Chantrix
Warfarin	Depo-provera
Diovan	Protonix
Crestor	Norvasc
Lisinopril	Benicar

Many people suffer with chronic back pain, neck pain, headaches, muscle and joint pain, and paresthesias, and they take some of these drugs. Others have chronic pain and don't take any of these pills.

Here's the point.

The drug information above is from conventional medical literature. All doctors have access to the drug information that says many forms of pain are caused by chemicals.

Chronic pain is not caused by physical trauma. Chronic pain is aggravated by physical trauma.

Chronic pain is a chemical phenomenon.

Chronic pain is caused by diet and drugs.

Pain can not be proven. Pain is anecdotal.

Here are some anecdotes.

Scoliosis does not cause back pain.

11. Some Stories

Debbie S. was a 52 year old yoga instructor who was in good shape. She had recurring neck pain. Debbie started experiencing lower back pain after she started taking lamictal for depression in September of 2009. She would not quit and saw an MD for the severe muscular pain that is clearly listed as one of the possible side effects of lamictal. The doctor prescribed Carispoprodol for pain. She took the first pill at 6pm on January 28, 2010 and died that night.

Headaches — Evista

Sandy S. was a 58 year old woman — Severe migraines began 4 days after starting Evista for osteoporosis. She stopped Evista on 4/9/03. She had headaches during the next 30 days after chocolate and MSG in Chinese food and flavored coffee creamer (caseinate). Her headaches were gone 33 days after she quit taking Evista.

Restless legs — Omeprazole

Lonnie W. 66 year old male had leg jumpies at night — omeprazole. (in prilosec, nexium, pepcid) His symptoms decreased dramatically when he quit omeprazole and switched to Tums™.

Sciatic pain — Zocor

Ronald O. had back pain and right leg pain for many years. He had a laminectomy in 2003 and felt no pain for 5 years, then his pain came back. He came in to see me on 9/29/09. He ate chocolate every day and had been taking Zocor for two years. We eliminated dairy and chocolate and zocor and he recovered in 96 days.

Sciatic pain — dairy foods

Virginia came in with severe sciatic pain that she had been suffering with for one year. She received treatment in my office for three weeks and eliminated all dairy foods from her diet. She recovered in 22 days.

Trigger finger — symvastatin/casein

One year later in August of 2010 Virginia came in with a flexion contracture of her middle finger on the left hand. It had been bothering her for a month. Each morning on rising her middle finger was flexed against the palm of her hand and it wouldn't move for several hours. She had been taking Symvastatin for two months. She stopped taking the statin drug and came in three times for physical therapy. She recovered in 7 days.

Virginia returned in January 2011 with a recurrence of her contracture that had been bothering her for two months. She was using a flavored creamer (containing caseinate) in her coffee for a few months. I had her change her coffee creamer to a soy milk and she recovered in 7 days.

Loss of peripheral vision — dairy foods.

John W. failed his truck driver's physical exam in my office because he had no peripheral vision in his right eye. He told me he suffered with right half-head migraines daily. I had him come in as a patient. He was a big milk drinker. I had him eliminate all dairy foods. Two weeks later he passed his exam and was headache free.

Psoriasis — dairy foods (see page 120)

Dave E. came in for migraines and right knee swelling. I had him take off his pants and his legs were covered with bright red, pepperoni sized red sores: psoriasis. I had him eliminate all dairy foods for his headaches. His headaches were eliminated, his knee swelling went away (also with therapy), and his psoriasis disappeared in 63 days.

Pain and dizziness — dairy, chocolate, MSG.

Debbra C. came into my office complaining of numbness in the lower back and legs, dizziness, headaches every day. These symptoms had been going on for two years. She consulted a medical doctor who referred her to a neurologist who told her it was not MS. He performed an EMG (worthless painful test, it never changes anything)

She loved milk and drank several glasses of whole milk every day. She ate cheese every day. She ate chocolate several times a week. She smoked a half a pack a day. She ate canned tuna two to three times a week. She put soy sauce on everything. I had her eliminate dairy foods, chocolate, and MSG. Within two weeks all of her symptoms were gone.

I agreed with the neurologist. It wasn't MS

Headaches — casein and MSG

Lily suffered with headaches for years. She worked at Kaiser where doctors told her it was stress — just relax, they said. Then one day while driving she ate a chocolate candy bar and immediately got a headache. She quit chocolate and her headaches stopped. She consulted me in June of 2008 for severe left hip and groin pain that she suffered with for three years. Kaiser doctors could find nothing wrong. Physical therapy didn't help.

We started treatment on 6/5/08 — took her off dairy, chocolate (already quit) and MSG. She recovered in 13 days, then had two recurrences — one after mashed potatoes in a restaurant (milk), and once again after Chinese food in a restaurant (MSG) — that also caused a headache.

Lower back pain — casein and gluten

Karen D. began treatment on 3/17/08 for lower back pain. She cancelled a vacation after one week of treatment because she was motivated to recover. Many patients quit my program in the first week if there is no progress. Her disciplined approach to my treatment plan was rare for a lupus patient. Three weeks later, after eliminating all dairy foods and chocolate, her condition had improved only slightly.

On 4/17/08 I had her eliminate all gluten from her diet. On 4/21/08 she came into the office and said, "We have lift off." Office visits ended on 5/09/08. Her medical doctor described her symptoms as Lupus. She described her symptoms as feeling congested. Her joints and muscles felt congested. Now she feels uncongested and free of pain. It took 60 days.

Dizziness — toporol, plavix, tenormin

Leota has been a patient for many years. In January of 2001 at the age of 73 her medical doctors decided she needed a pace maker. In 2004 her doctors prescribed **toporol** and she immediately began experiencing dizziness. She couldn't walk without hanging on to the walls. She quit toporol due to dizziness and nose bleeds, but her doctors insisted on other meds. She was on **plavix**, then **tenormin**. Her dizziness persisted. In October of 2005 I wrote in my chart notes that I felt her dizziness was due to meds, but her doctors insisted, and scared her into believing that she couldn't stop taking them. In July of 2006 she suffered a TIA (transient ischemic attack) and was rushed to the hospital immediately by her daughter, an RN. They released her a few hours later and she went home and suffered a full blown stroke the following day. She lost

139

feeling and muscle control of her right arm and leg. In August her daughter insisted the doctor consider her medication. He told her to stop all of them. Her dizziness is now gone, after being the main complaint in her life for six years.

Knee pain — Xanax

Cindy M. has been a patient for many years. She and her husband are team truck drivers and have been driving over the road together for ten years. In 2004 they began working for an auto transport company delivering cars to dealerships. Part of their job involved climbing up on the trailer, into cars, then driving them down the ramps to the ground. Likewise when loading the cars, they had to climb down off the trailer after they secured each car they loaded.

On 12/3/04 Cindy came into my office complaining of low back pain, and bilateral knee pain that had begun in the last month. The logical conclusion was that the pain was due to all the climbing, and that was probably part of her case. But she had been doing the job for many months before the knee pain began.

After starting this new job earlier in the year, Cindy became nervous about the work, the pay, etc., and she began experiencing panic attacks. She consulted a medical doctor who prescribed **xanax**. She started taking xanax in mid October, and her knee pain began two weeks later. We decided to cut her dose of xanax in half. By 12/23/04 her knee pain was gone.

Side effects to xanax in order:

Fatigue	13.9%
Depression	12.1
Dry mouth	10.2
Constipation	8.0
Appetite up or down	7.0
Decreased libido	6.0
Dysmennorhea	3.6
Arthralgia	**2.4**
Sexual Dysfunction	2.4

Other side affects include runny nose, hot flashes, road traffic accident, influenza, and the ever popular paresthesias.

Mitt hand — avandia and glipizide

Joe B. was 82 and came into my office on 1/19/01. His right hand looked like a baseball mitt. His left hand looked normal, but he complained of pain and weakness in both hands, worse on the right. He had consulted his medical doctor who referred him to a specialist who told Joe that he had carpal tunnel and that his nerves were all jangled up in his wrist. Maybe "jangled up" was Joe's translation, but it reminds me of an episode many years ago when one of my patients was taken away and sent to a specialist who spent a day and several thousands of dollars in tests to arrive at his assessment of her back pain: "Honey," he said, "you have wrenched your back."

For the life of me. I didn't see a wrench in my x-ray or in his.

I tested Joe's grip strength. Although Joe is right handed, he did not move the needle with his right hand. He gripped 70 pounds with his left hand.

It was my opinion, as unspecialized as it is, that his nerves were not all jangled up. I told him he had a form of paresthesia

141

and neuropathy that would require physical therapy and diet manipulation. Joe was a diabetic and was taking **glipizide** and **avandia**. He monitored his blood sugar daily, and reported that it ran between 190 and 250 — still too high. His doctor's response to Joe's high blood sugar was to increase the dose of both drugs. Despite taking the medication, Joe had all the signs of diabetes. He had to get out of bed six to seven times a night to urinate.

Joe was a big milk drinker and dairy user, so I decided we could fix him up with the elimination of dairy (casein) along with a series of treatments on his wrists and hands. After two weeks of therapy, Joe was following the diet strictly, but had failed to respond. However, he reported that within one week of no dairy foods, he was down to one to two trips to the toilet at night. His blood sugar was still around 200.

On 1/29/01, Joe was depressed about his progress. Although his sugar was still testing high, I instructed him to stop the glipizide and avandia. On 2/3/01, his blood sugar was 230. On 2/5/01 it dropped to 183, and two days later on 2/7/01, it was 146. On 2/3 and 2/4/01 he did not get up at night to urinate. His hand had failed to respond.

On 2/9/01 I discovered that we had a communication problem. He had discontinued only one of his pills, the glipizide, but was still taking avandia. Per my instructions, he discontinued the avandia on 2/9/01.

Once Joe was off both avandia and glipizide, the swelling in his right hand diminished very rapidly. By 2/28/01, three weeks after stopping these pills, Joe's hand looked normal, no swelling, and worked well. The PDR lists many side affects for glipizide and avandia including paresthesia, pain, myalgia, arhralgia, polyuria, swelling, leg cramps, and blurred vision.

Low back pain — lipitor

Joe was released at that time, but returned three years later with lower back pain. This pain had begun two months after his doctors started him on **lipitor** for high cholesterol. He received three treatments which included spinal manipulation, physical therapy, and the elimination of lipitor. He recovered and was released.

Statin drugs are the worst pills on the market today, for several reasons. These drugs are used to address the cholesterol issue, which most doctors today view as a critical measure of a patient's ability to keep from falling over dead. Many doctors today believe that any cholesterol reading that is not low normal, requires medication. This aggressive attitude by M.D.s today has driven Lipitor to become the number two most prescribed drug in the country (after vicodin for pain).

I began witnessing musculoskeletal problems caused by cholesterol drugs in 2000. I read *The People's Pharmacy* column in the L.A. Times on July 14, 2000 in which a woman witnessed her husband's back problems that began after he started taking Zocor. She wrote : "All of his doctors, without exception, insist that his back pain could not be related to Mevocor or Zocor." But when the doctors were forced to stop Zocor when he showed signs of liver damage, his pain went away.

The most common side effects I have seen are leg pain and weakness, foot and lower leg numbness and pain, low back pain, and sciatic pain.

The statin drugs are so powerful and potentially harmful that liver and kidney tests must be performed every few months. When these vital organs begin to fail, the medication is stopped. But many of the patients I see receive only a few tests in the first few months, then they proceed with the statins, unchecked, for years. On the TV commercial, the warning is played down: "Simple blood tests may be necessary to check for kidney of liver problems." The tests may be simple, but the organ problems are not.

Many patients who are instructed by me to immediately stop these pills react with confusion and doubt. "I might die."

I assure them they won't die from not taking statin drugs. They will just feel better.

But then they come back from that fateful visit to the M.D. who has put the scare into them. "You *must* take these drugs or you will die!" (that's an actual quote. Another one is, "Ok, go ahead and die.")

The persistent patients are usually berated by their M.D.'s. When a health care practitioner tells a patient they will die if they don't take statin drugs, they are no longer practicing health care. When I recommend the elimination of statin drugs, about half the patients continue with the drugs, and about half of them follow my instructions. Most of the patients who quit have a full recovery.

Recovery times vary from a few days to six months. In some cases, the symptoms are irreversible, and the patients do not recover from the damage done by statins.

I have talked to many patients who stopped the statin drugs on their own when they felt worse for taking them. I have also talked to patients who were already informed about the dangers of the statins, and refused to even start taking them.

Back in 2000, I had seen several patients respond to the elimination of statins before I read the article mentioned above. After reading that article, I copied it and framed it and placed one in each of my treatment rooms.

Calf weakness — zocor

Don M. was 76 and came in for leg weakness in both calves. He had failed to list Zocor as one of his medications, but read the article on the wall after two weeks of treatment. He told me he was taking Zocor, we agreed to stop the Zocor, and his leg weakness disappeared in two weeks.

Liver pain and yellow eyes — lipitor

Louise W. has seen me for years for various back problems, mainly upper back pain that is recurring due to a botched arm surgery that left her right arm with no bony attachment to her torso. After consulting her M.D. a few months ago, she was prescribed lipitor. After taking it for two months, her sister came over for a visit and noticed that the whites of her eyes were yellow. Louise then told her of her pain in the right upper abdomen where her liver is located. Calls to her doctor were not returned, so she called the pharmacist and related the story to him. He instructed her to immediately stop taking lipitor.

The statin drugs often cause liver and kidney damage. Like the commercials say, "simple tests are required to check for liver damage." The tests may be simple, but liver damage is not so simple. Many doctors have become so complacent about prescribing statins that they no longer order periodic liver tests. This is extremely dangerous. Of course, the argument by the makers of these drugs, again like the TV commercials point out, these side effects are "rare but serious" problems.

None of the patients mentioned above have reported their problems to the drug companies. These side effects are not nearly as rare as the makers would have you believe. But millions of people take these drugs, and even in the best case scenario, thousands of them will suffer with side effects. The one or two percent that are documented don't include the many, many people who have discovered on their own that they felt terrible after taking statin drugs. Any patient who hasn't been scared to death by his doctor would immediately stop these terrible and unnecessary drugs if they felt any of the misery that I have seen in my office.

Hair loss and joint pain — Lipitor

Merri D. took Lipitor for two weeks. During that time her hair began to fall out by the handful and she had severe joint pain, mainly in her hips. She quit Lipitor on her own and her symptoms stopped.

Linda H. told me the same story on the same day: she had hair loss and severe lower back pain immediately after starting lipitor. She quit and the pain and hair loss stopped.

Elizabeth came into my office in 2008 complaining of left leg pain and cramps. She had been taking zocor for six years and ate dairy foods every day — organic milk. A medical doctor told her that her leg pain was "probably arthritis". She was diabetic and took metformin. I instructed her to stop dairy foods and zocor.

She recovered. She came back on February 28, 2011 with the same complaints, but worse. She described severe burning pain in her hip and left leg. Her drug list had expanded to include 12 drugs.

Her pain was now due to a work injury in 2009. Lots of drugs included insulin, metformin, januvia, and prandin for diabetes.. She was now on Gemfibrozil for cholesterol.

Her voice was raspy and her leg pain was severe.

Gemfibrozil was a new one for me, so I looked it up. It was not to be taken with prandin, which she was taking.

Listed as a rare side effect to prandin was hoarseness. Elizabeth had that and sometimes could be barely understood. People thought she was mentally challenged.

My instructions were for her to quit dairy foods and Gemfibrozil. She quit prandin on her own. Her voice was normal in 29 days. Her hip pain diminished gradually.

Sciatic pain — dairy foods

Maria first came to see me in January on 2007 complaining of severe right leg pain. She could barely walk. She was 84 years old and, amazingly, was taking no medication. On January 3, 2007 we began treatment with chiropractic care and physical therapy and we had her stop consuming dairy foods. She was using milk on cereal daily, and cheese three to four times a week. After many ups and downs, she recovered and was released on February 20, 2007, 17 days after quitting all casein in dairy foods..

She returned two months later on 4/25/07 with severe left shoulder pain. She could not raise her arm above her waist. After examining her and questioning her, we began a course of physical therapy, home exercises, and the elimination of the cheese that she had begun eating two or three times a week for the last two weeks — just before her shoulder pain began. She completely recovered after four treatments and was released on May 1, 2007, six days.

Shoulder pain — Activia™

Maria returned again on 6/14/07 with the same severe left shoulder pain. She was avoiding all dairy foods (we thought, at first). Her daughter always accompanied her to the office, and she spoke better English, so I asked her about dairy foods. She told me they were using soy milk on cereal and avoiding all dairy foods. When I asked her if her mother was taking any new medications, she said she had started taking **Activia™** two weeks ago.

She presumed it was some sort of medication, because she saw it advertised on TV as a healthy thing to take for overall general health. Activia™ is yogurt and contains casein. I instructed her to stop using Activia™ and Maria recovered with two treatments.

Activia™ is advertised on prime time TV as some sort of miracle health adjunct. Because of the presentation, Maria's daughter failed to consider that it was just yogurt, a dairy food. She thought it would do her mother some good, because they said so on TV.

Belching — dairy foods

Ricardo was 60 years old when he came to see me on 6/4/07. He was suffering with neck pain, shoulder pain, right arm and hand pain, headaches, and lower back pain. When I came into the room with him, my first observation was his constant belching.

We began our discussion about his digestive symptoms because they were so graphic. Ricardo was belching every 5 seconds. He had seen MD's for all of the above conditions. Pain pills, x-rays and CT scans had changed nothing and failed to answer the question: what is wrong with Ricardo? He tried **pepcid** for a few months, no change. He belched all the time. Now he was trying **omeprazole**, beginning the day he first saw me. I told him not to bother with the omeprazole.

Ricardo is an amazingly compliant patient. He was a regular dairy user (milk on cereal 3-4X a week, cheese 2-3X a week. He ate out at restaurants 2-3X a week.) I instructed him to stop using all dairy foods, chocolate, and MSG. On 6/14/07, after ten days, the headaches were gone. He belched once on 6/14/07, then not again until 7/24/07.

He was coming in twice a week for adjustments and physical therapy. His overall condition improved a lot — no more headaches, no digestive problems, and his neck and back pain were less — but still there. He had slipped on the diet two times: once reacting to turkey sausage (MSG) with a headache, then another headache on 7/19/07 after barley soup at a restaurant (MSG).

On 6/28/07 we added gluten (wheat) to his list of foods to avoid. From 6/28/07 to 7/24/07 there was no change in his condition. He still had neck pain and stiffness, right arm pain, and lower back pain. On 7/24/07 he awoke with severe stomach and back pain. He had been good on the diet, and on 7/23/07 he ate chicken and rice, as usual. Two hours later he ate a lot of jello that contained gelatin and aspartame. This was the first jello he had eaten since we started treatment.

In further questioning about his diet, it was revealed that he was chewing sugar free gum nearly every day because his breath was so bad. On 7/26/07 I gave Ricardo a more extensive list of MSG names which included Gelatin as a food that always contains MSG. I instructed him to stop chewing gum.

Ricardo still has lots of problems, but avoiding dairy, chocolate, gluten, MSG, and aspartame have improved his condition immensely.

Back pain, weakness — Benicar

Ray has a lifetime work comp case. He has a recurring low back problem, and once a year, or so, he comes in for treatment when his back and right sciatic pain bother him. He was taking no medication. This year he came in with his same problem, along with severe weakness and shortness of breath, chest pain, and swelling in the ankles. He had gone back to using some dairy foods and MSG, so we got him back on track with his diet, and did some treatment. After three weeks, he failed to improve. He then remembered that he had started taking **Benicar**, for blood pressure, nine months earlier. After four weeks of treatment, I was about to give up. I told him to go see his MD for more tests. But before he left, I took his blood pressure. It was 90/60 — way too low. I instructed him to stop taking Benicar, and within 10 days, his blood pressure was up to normal and his pain was gone. The PDR (Physician's Desk Reference) lists arthritis, arthralgia (joint pain), chest pain, peripheral edema, and myalgia (muscle pain) as possible side-effects to Benicar.

Sciatic pain — dairy, chocolate, MSG

Bonnie came in to see me in 2006 for left sciatic pain that had plagued her for a year. We fixed her up with chiropractic care and the elimination of dairy foods in six weeks. She had several recurrences in the next year when she went back to eating dairy foods. Her pain was also aggravated by MSG.

She returned to the office again in 2008 because, despite our success with her sciatic pain, Bonnie still complained of severe left foot pain and spasms, especially at night, and more so after a long day of work on her feet. She was still off dairy foods and MSG. I asked her about her medications, and she was taking none, except an herbal concoction for hormone replacement. I instructed her to discontinue the Herbal Replacement Therapy by Natural Max, and her foot pain subsided and was gone in 5 weeks. Her supplement contained Peruvian Maca, Soy, black cohosh, dong quai, red clover and pomegranate. The herbal concoction is encapsulated in a gelatin capsule, which, according to Russell Blaylock, M.D., contains free glutamate.

Leg cramps — lisinopril

Janet R. had leg cramps for one month. Her doctor had prescribed **benzapril** two years ago to control her blood pressure. After one year he wasn't satisfied, so he changed her to 10mg. of **Lisinopril** in 4/07. In 2/08 he upped the dose to 40mg. of Lisinopril. On about 3/23/07 she began getting severe leg cramps at night. She could not sleep. On 4/23/08 Janet and I agreed that she should stop taking the Lisinopril. Her leg cramps stopped in two days and have not returned.

Shoulder and arm pain — salted cashews (MSG)

Tom was a sixty five year old left handed softball player when he first saw me in 2004 for left shoulder pain. We had him eliminate dairy foods and he received four treatments in seven days and he recovered.

He came in again five years later after he fell on his left shoulder playing ball. This time he had shoulder pain and severely decreased range of motion. He had trouble raising his arm, and he couldn't throw overhand. He was still off dairy foods, using soy milk on his cereal. In the interim he had lost 60 pounds. We did therapy for two months from January to March. His condition gradually improved until the end of March when suddenly both of his arms started to ache and his improvement ceased. He continued with therapy even though his progress was minimal until the beginning of May when he theorized that his pain had been worse since he began eating salted cashews every day. He quit them on 5/10/09. His right arm pain was completely gone in two days, and his left arm was 80% improved.

Back spasms — tricor

Gayle B. began experiencing severe mid back spasms after taking **Tricor** for two months. The spasms were gone within two days of quitting tricor.

Paula Z. came in on 2/15/11 complaining of severe teeth pain, headaches, and vision problems. The pain in her teeth was severe and began after braces on her teeth ten years ago. Several dentists and orthodontists, and a trigeminal nerve specialist all had no answers and resorted to medication.

Her daily meds included: Klonipin (for one year), nortryptalene (seven years), and advil.

She also took atenelol for blood pressure, and levothyroid.

She ate dairy foods regularly, and chocolate every day: cupcakes in the morning, Ovaltine™ at night.

She used Accent™ (pure MSG) in all of her cooking.

She stopped all dairy, chocolate, and MSG on 2/15/2011

She suffered with the pain off and on for about 14 days. She suffered withdrawal symptoms when she quit the advil on day 15 — headaches.

On day 28 she quit nortryptalene and suffered with severe body aches for 6 days.

From day 1 (2/15) to day 30 (3/17) she went from severe pain to felling "pretty darn good."

Eczema — milk allergy

Jay came in for a truck driver's physical and saw my book and the pictures of Dave's psoriasis (page 120) on the wall. He asked a few questions and bought a book. Two months later he came in and bought 12 books. He wanted to give books to others who had health problems.

He told me that his five year old daughter had suffered with eczema since birth. She scratched her dry, scaly arms until they bled. Her parents would take turns during the night rubbing lotion on her bloody arms. Within a few weeks of eliminating dairy foods, her condition has totally cleared.

12. Show and Tell

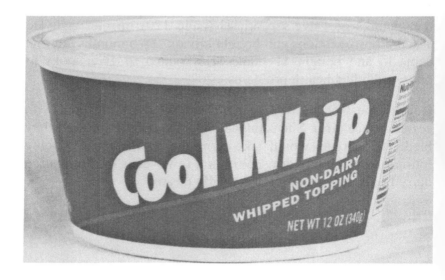

Cool Whip is called non-dairy...

INGREDIENTS: WATER, HYDROGENATED VEGETABLE OILS (COCONUT AND PALM KERNEL OILS), CORN SYRUP, HIGH FRUCTOSE CORN SYRUP, SUGAR, SODIUM CASEINATE (A MILK DERIVED INGREDIENT), LESS THAN ONE PERCENT OF NATURAL AND ARTIFICIAL FLAVORS, POLYSORBATE 60 AND SORBITAN MONOSTEARATE (FOR UNIFORM DISPERSION OF OIL), XANTHAN GUM AND GUAR GUM (THICKENERS), BETA CAROTENE (FOR COLOR).

But the label includes "sodium caseinate (a milk derived ingredient)

"Non-Dairy" is a legal term, not an accurate term.

Any product like a sauce, dressing mix, dip, or soup mix most likely contains MSG.

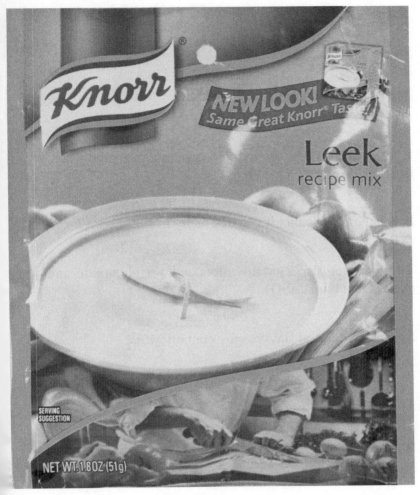

Knorr uses MSG in nearly all of their products. I haven't found one that doesn't contain some MSG.

See the label that follows.

INGREDIENTS: WHEAT FLOUR, MALTODEXTRIN, ONION POWDER, DEHYDRATED VEGETABLES (POTATOES, LEEKS), MODIFIED POTATO STARCH, SALT, HYDROLYZED CORN PROTEIN, MONOSODIUM GLUTAMATE, PARTIALLY HYDROGENATED SOYBEAN OIL, WHEY (MILK), GUAR GUM, YEAST EXTRACT, SPICES, NATURAL FLAVORS, TURMERIC, DISODIUM GUANYLATE, DISODIUM INOSINATE.

Hydrolyzed protein of any kind contains free glutamate, which is MSG.

In this Knorr product it is listed as hydrolyzed corn protein.

This product also contains monosodium glutamate and yeast extract (contains MSG).

Spices and natural flavors *may* contain MSG.

Any seasoning packet is suspect, especially when the label makes claims about flavor, like

"Great New Flavor"

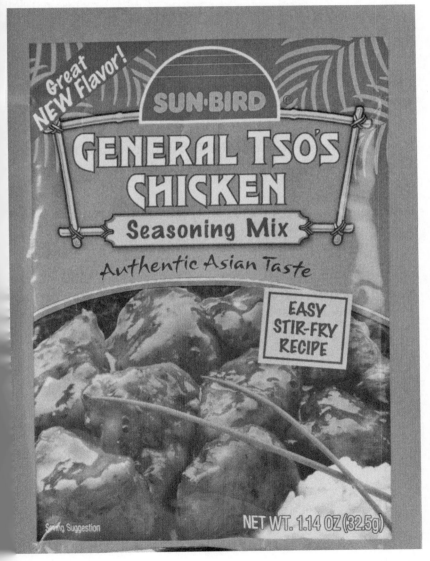

INGREDIENTS: MODIFIED CORN STARCH, DEHYDRATED GARLIC AND ONION, WHITE WINE POWDER (MALTODEXTRIN, DISTILLED WHITE WINE), SPICES, MONOSODIUM GLUTAMATE, NATURAL FLAVORS (YEAST EXTRACT), SALT, SODIUM DIACETATE, CITRIC ACID, CHICKEN FAT, LACTOSE (MILK), CARAMEL COLOR. CONTAINS: MILK

The flavor of any chicken dish will be great and new when monosodium glutamate and yeast extract are added.

It is difficult to create a chicken dish as tasty as one with MSG. You have to be clever with spices, and spend more money.

Restaurants want to provide tasty dishes that will keep you coming back.

Most restaurants are very liberal with their use of MSG instead of all the expensive spices and homemade spices that would taste as good, or great and new.

According to Dr. George Schwartz in his geat book, "In Bad Taste, The MSG Syndrome" salad dressings are the food type that most likely contains MSG.

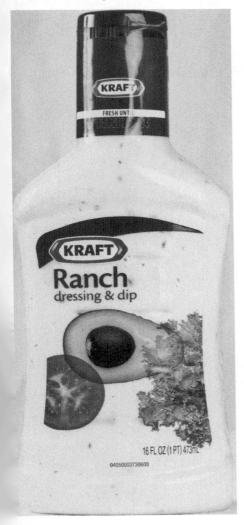

INGREDIENTS: WATER, SOYBEAN OIL, SUGAR, GARLIC JUICE, BUTTERMILK, CONTAINS LESS THAN 2% OF SALT, MODIFIED FOOD STARCH, WHEY, PHOSPHORIC ACID, MONOSODIUM GLUTAMATE, EGG WHITES, VINEGAR, XANTHAN GUM, CITRIC ACID, POLYSORBATE 60, SPICE, NATURAL FLAVOR, ENZYMES, WITH SODIUM LACTATE, NATAMYCIN, AND CALCIUM DISODIUM EDTA AS PRESERVATIVES

CONTAINS: MILK, EGG.

Ranch dressing contains dairy (buttermilk) and MSG.

Caesar dressing always contains parmesan cheese, one of the most powerful forms of casein. Parmesan cheese is a dried cheese, containing less water, and a higher concentration of casein.

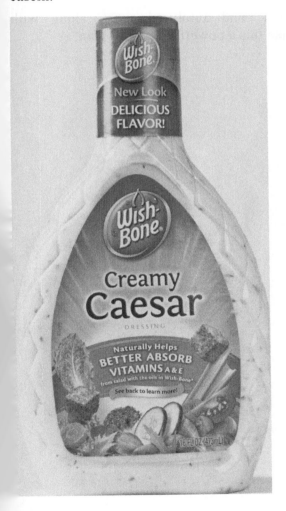

INGREDIENTS: SOYBEAN OIL, WATER, DISTILLED VINEGAR, EGG YOLKS, SUGAR, PARMESAN CHEESE (MILK, CHEESE CULTURES, SALT, ENZYMES), SALT, ANCHOVIES (FISH), SOY SAUCE (WATER, WHEAT, SOYBEANS, SALT), GARLIC, SPICES, PHOSPHORIC ACID, ONION, MONOSODIUM GLUTAMATE, SORBIC ACID AND SODIUM BENZOATE AND CALCIUM DISODIUM EDTA (USED TO PROTECT QUALITY), CORN SYRUP, POLYSORBATE 60, XANTHAN GUM, GARLIC POWDER, SOY FLOUR, AUTOLYZED YEAST EXTRACT, NATURAL AND ARTIFICIAL FLAVORS, TAMARIND.

Monosodium glutamate and autolyzed yeast, along with parmesan cheese, make this a powerful cause of pain.

Dip mixes are supposed to add flavor.

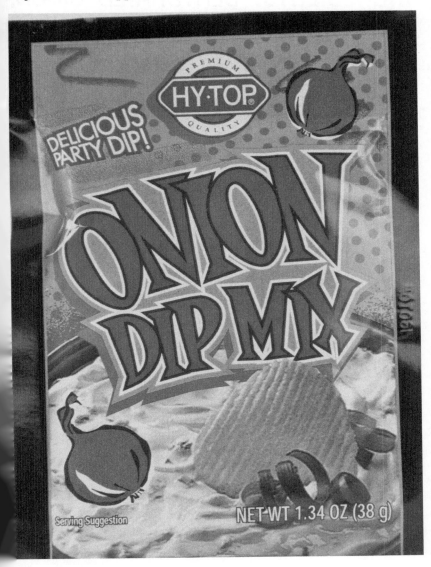

This is a packet (suspect MSG)

INGREDIENTS: DEHYDRATED ONION, SALT, WHEAT STARCH, MONOSODIUM GLUTAMATE, DEXTROSE, TORULA YEAST, HYDROLYZED SOY PROTEIN, PARTIALLY HYDROGENATED SOYBEAN/COTTONSEED OILS, YEAST EXTRACT, SUGAR, SILICON DIOXIDE (ANTI-CAKE), CARAMEL COLOR, MALTODEXTRIN, NATURAL FLAVORS, DISODIUM INOSINATE, DISODIUM GUANYLATE.

Look for the ingredients with lots of x's and y's, and names you can't pronounce.

Monosodium glutamate, hydrolyzed protein, and yeast extract are three sources of MSG and make this a very powerful and tasty dish that is toxic to your nervous system.

Here's a packet from McCormick that checks off No MSG for you.

But what's that little † symbol after MSG?

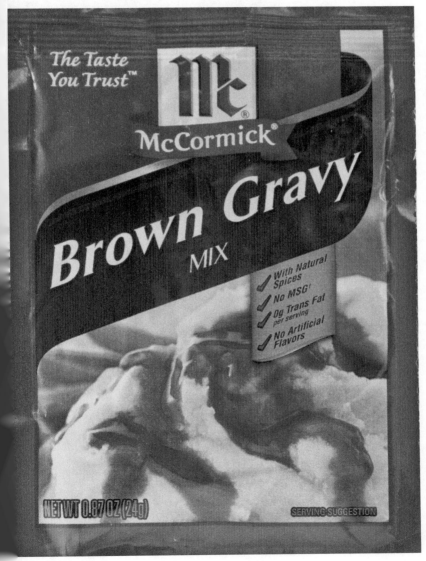

Here's the label.

INGREDIENTS: ENRICHED WHEAT FLOUR (FLOUR, NIACIN, IRON, THIAMINE MONO-NITRATE, RIBOFLAVIN, FOLIC ACID), WHEAT STARCH, SALT, BEEF FAT, HYDROLYZED SOY, WHEAT AND CORN PROTEIN, ONION, CARAMEL COLOR, CORN SYRUP SOLIDS, SPICES, SODIUM CASEINATE (MILK), GARLIC, WHEAT PROTEIN, DISODIUM INOSINATE AND DISODIUM GUANYLATE (FLAVOR ENHANCERS), EXTRACTIVES OF PAPRIKA, YEAST EXTRACT, AND CITRIC ACID.

Yeast extract and sodium caseinate (dairy) are ingredients in this product.

According to Russell Blaylock, M.D., in his book, *Excitotoxins: The Taste that Kills*, sodium caseinate is not only dairy, but also a source of free glutamate found in MSG.

This McCormick ad for their taco seasoning (another packet = warning!), also boasts No MSG†.

Get out your magnifying glass.

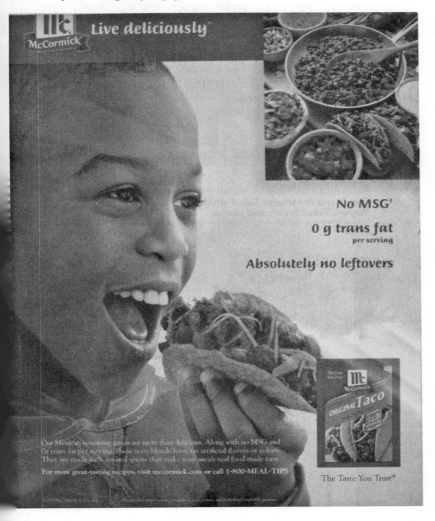

See the small print at the bottom?

No, the smaller print way at the bottom of the page.

Check out the very, very, very small print at the bottom.

†Except that which occurs naturally in yeast extract and hydrolyzed vegetable proteins.

The taste you trust uses the smallest print possible, there at the bottom:

"except that which occurs naturally in yeast extract and hydrolyzed vegetable protein."

Do you think they wanted you to know that?

Their label says "No MSG," but their product contains MSG.

Here's another misleading label by Swanson's.

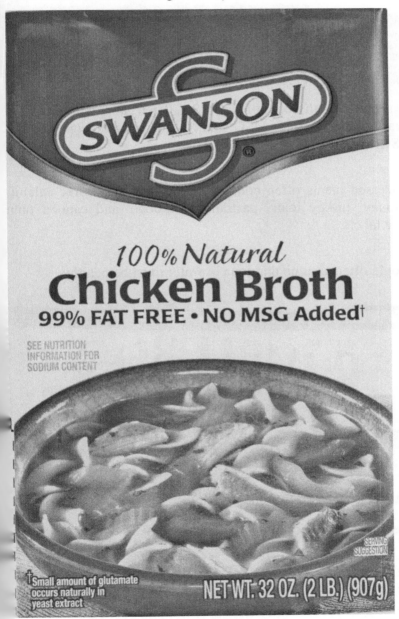

Check out the bottom left corner of their box. Here is the label:

INGREDIENTS: CHICKEN STOCK, CONTAINS LESS THAN 2% OF: SEA SALT, SALT, NATURAL FLAVORING, SUGAR, DEHYDRATED ONIONS, YEAST EXTRACT, CHICKEN FAT, CARROTS, CELERY, ONIONS.

Swanson's broth does contain MSG. Their label is misleading. Yeast extract contains MSG, and Natural Flavors *might* contain MSG.

Processed meats often contain MSG. Deli meats like salami, boloney, turkey loafs, pastrami, hot dogs, and canned tuna have labels.

People often assume that tuna in water must be healthy.

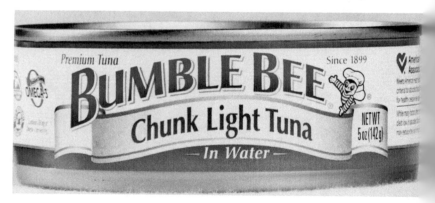

But most canned tuna contains MSG.

Check out the list of ingredients that follows.

INGREDIENTS: LIGHT TUNA, WATER, VEGETABLE BROTH, SALT
CONTAINS: TUNA, SOY

DISTRIBUTED BY:
©BUMBLE BEE FOODS, LLC
SAN DIEGO, CA 92186 USA
www.bumblebee.com
MAY CONTAIN BONES

Vegetable broth contains MSG.

However, Bumble Bee also carries tuna that does not contain MSG. Low sodium tuna is a healthy alternative, and it usually does not contain MSG.

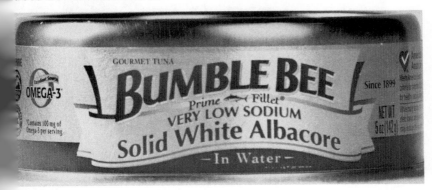

This product contains no MSG.

See?

They should advertise "No MSG" on their label.

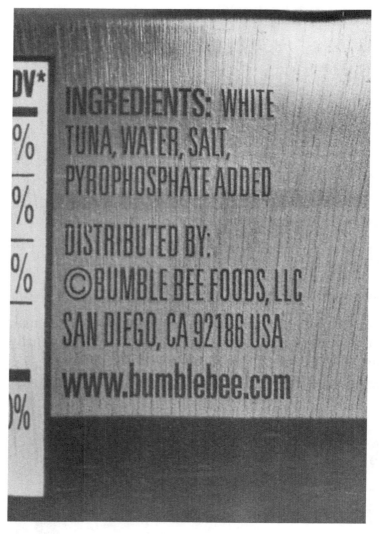

No MSG (pyrophosphate is a preservative)

Sometimes low sodium tuna, or diet tuna, is found on the diet aisle of the grocery store.

Canned salmon does not contain MSG (usually).

Bologna (or baloney) is a heavily processed meat food, both chemically (and mechanically? Poor animals) and contains MSG.

This bologna has a first name and a last name and it's Oscar Mayer. Name brands, like Oscar Mayer, usually use less MSG. But the cheaper brands, like Carl Buddig® and store brands tend to use more MSG.

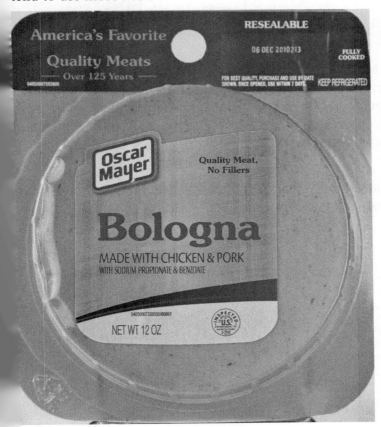

INGREDIENTS: MECHANICALLY SEPARATED CHICKEN, PORK, WATER, CORN SYRUP, CONTAINS LESS THAN 2% OF SALT, GROUND MUSTARD SEED, SODIUM PHOSPHATES, AUTOLYZED YEAST, SODIUM PROPIONATE, POTASSIUM CHLORIDE, SODIUM DIACETATE, SODIUM BENZOATE, SODIUM ASCORBATE, SODIUM NITRITE, FLAVOR, EXTRACTIVES OF PAPRIKA, OLEORESIN CELERY SEED, POTASSIUM PHOSPHATE.

Oscar Mayer may contain less MSG than other brands, but this product still contains autolyzed yeast — a nerve toxin that contributes to, or causes pain and chronic pain when these heavily processed foods are a regular part of the Standard American Diet (SAD).

Look at all the other ingredients listed in this product that obviously did not grow on a tree.

174

Almost all sausage contains MSG.

Hillshire Farm products use lots of MSG.

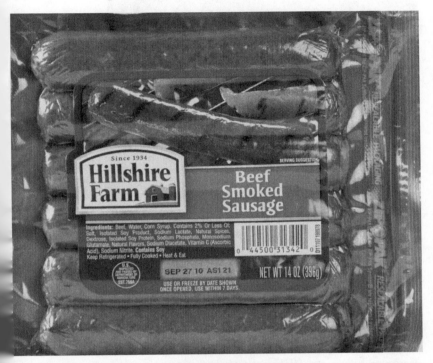

Ingredients: Beef, Water, Corn Syrup, Contains 2% Or Less Of: Salt, Isolated Soy Product, Sodium Lactate, Natural Spices, Dextrose, Isolated Soy Protein, Sodium Phosphate, Monosodium Glutamate, Natural Flavors, Sodium Diacetate, Vitamin C (Ascorbic Acid), Sodium Nitrite. **Contains Soy**
Keep Refrigerated • Fully Cooked • Heat & Eat

This product includes monosodium glutamate by name. But any protein isolate, or isolated protein also contains MSG.

Protein isolate is one of the first five ingredients in most protein shakes. This one is whey protein, no casein, but…

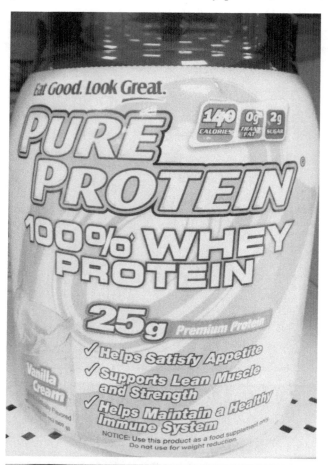

Ingredients: Protein Blend (Ultrafiltered Whey Protein Concentrate [which contains Beta-lactoglobulin, Alpha-lactalbumin and Glycomacropeptides], Microfiltered Whey Protein Isolate), Natural and Artificial Flavors, Cellulose Gum, Soy Lecithin, Xanthan Gum, Dicalcium Phosphate, Calcium Carbonate, Acesulfame Potassium, Sucralose. Contains milk and soy ingredients.
Contents...

Protein isolate, starting way at the right side and finishing on the next line at left, contains free glutamate, a nerve toxin.

This can of Campbell's Healthy request Soup is now available.

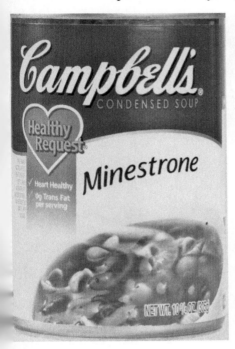

It contains MSG.

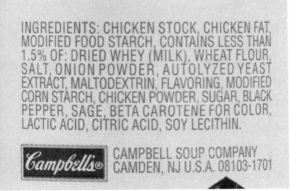

The chicken stock, flavoring, and the chicken powder likely contain MSG. Autolyzed yeast contains MSG

This is an older can that has been discontinued.

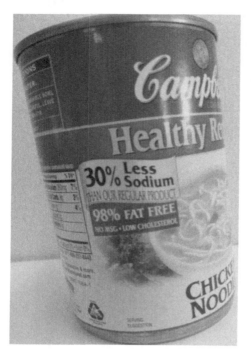

This one actually advertises "No MSG" right there below "98% Fat Free."

I used to recommend this soup for years, but it is no longer available.

I know of no canned soup that does not contain MSG.

Almost all restaurants use MSG in their soups.

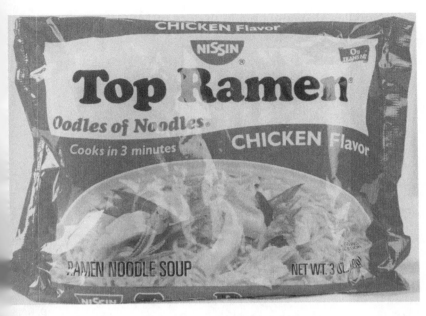

Dried soup mixes contain **high doses** of MSG.

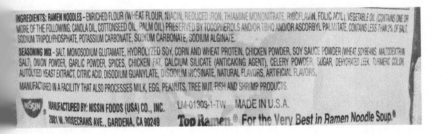

The second ingredient (meaning the second most stuff in this packet after salt) in the seasoning mix is MSG. The noodles, while highly processed, contain no MSG until the packet is added. This cheap food is widely popular.

Kids and inmates consume tons of this stuff.

Cup Noodles also contain a high dose of MSG.

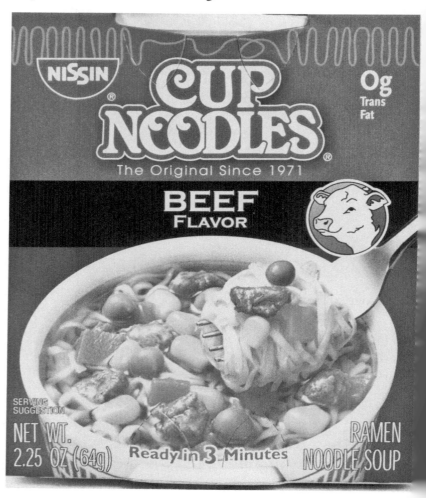

The label follows.

INGREDIENTS: ENRICHED WHEAT FLOUR (WHEAT FLOUR, NIACIN, REDUCED IRON, THIAMINE MONONITRATE, RIBOFLAVIN, FOLIC ACID), VEGETABLE OIL (PALM OIL, CANOLA OIL, PARTIALLY HYDROGENATED COTTONSEED AND SOYBEAN OIL, RICE BRAN OIL), SALT, TEXTURED SOY PROTEIN, CONTAINS LESS THAN 2% OF DRIED CARROT FLAKE, HYDROLYZED SOY PROTEIN, DRIED CORN, DRIED GREEN PEA, MONOSODIUM GLUTAMATE, ONION POWDER, CORN SYRUP, CARAMEL COLOR, GARLIC POWDER, HYDROLYZED CORN PROTEIN, POTASSIUM CARBONATE, SODIUM CARBONATE, SODIUM TRIPOLYPHOSPHATE, AUTOLYZED YEAST EXTRACT, DISODIUM GUANYLATE, DISODIUM INOSINATE, CITRIC ACID, NATURAL FLAVOR, BEEF FAT, BAKER'S YEAST EXTRACT, GELATIN, TBHQ (PRESERVATIVE), POWDERED BEEF, SODIUM ALGINATE, SUGAR, HYDROLYZED WHEAT PROTEIN, SOY SAUCE (WATER, WHEAT, SOYBEAN, SALT).

CONTAINS WHEAT AND SOYBEAN.

MANUFACTURED IN A FACILITY THAT PROCESSES MILK, EGG, PEANUT, TREE NUTS, CRUSTACEAN SHELLFISH, AND FISH PRODUCTS.

 MANUFACTURED BY: NISSIN FOODS (USA) CO., INC.
2001 W. ROSECRANS AVE., GARDENA, CA 90249

Any label with this many ingredients is an extremely processed food….and it contains lots of MSG.

Hydrolyzed soy protein, yeast extract, autolyzed yeast extract, gelatin, monosodium glutamate, and more are multiple sources of MSG.

This is what your kids are eating at school.

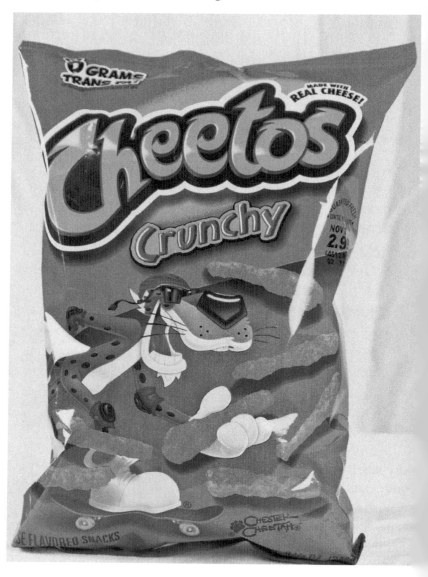

Ingredients: Enriched Corn Meal (Corn Meal, Ferrous Sulfate, Niacin, Thiamin Mononitrate, Riboflavin, and Folic Acid), Vegetable Oil (Contains One or More of the Following: Corn, Soybean, or Sunflower Oil), Cheese Seasoning (Whey, Cheddar Cheese [Milk, Cheese Cultures, Salt, Enzymes], and Less Than 2% of the Following: Partially Hydrogenated Soybean Oil, Salt, Maltodextrin, Disodium Phosphate, Sour Cream [Cultured Cream, Nonfat Milk], Artificial Flavor, Monosodium Glutamate, Lactic Acid, Artificial Color [Including Yellow 6], Citric Acid), and Salt.
CONTAINS MILK INGREDIENTS.

This product contains lots of MSG. This powerful nerve toxin contributes to and causes teenage neuro-funk, like attention deficit, learning disorders, depression, mood changes, panic attacks, and more.

Lots of dairy ingredients, and a powerful dose of MSG are included in this bag.

All flavored snack foods contain MSG to add flavoring. Plain chips, like Lays and Ruffles, plain Doritos, plain Pringles, plain Fritos, etc., have no MSG.

183

Regular rice, white and brown, contain no MSG.

But Rice-a-Roni has more…

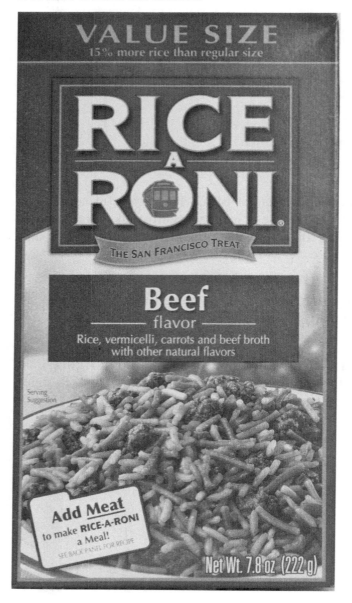

Ingredients: Rice, wheat flour, durum wheat semolina, salt, onions*, hydrolyzed protein (corn, soy and wheat), carrots*, sugar, monosodium glutamate, caramel color, beef broth*, natural flavor, garlic*, autolyzed yeast extract*, hydrolyzed gluten (wheat and corn) and hydrolyzed soy protein, disodium inosinate, niacin, disodium guanylate, ferric orthophosphate, ferrous sulfate, thiamin mononitrate, milk, folic acid, riboflavin. *Dried.
CONTAINS WHEAT, SOY AND MILK INGREDIENTS.

Rice-a-Roni has lots of MSG: hydrolyzed proteins (several), autolyzed yeast, beef broth, and monosodium glutamate.

TV Dinners all contain MSG, even Lean Cuisine.

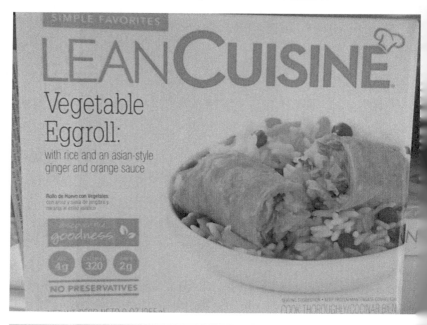

INGREDIENTS: VEGETABLE EGG ROLL (FILLING INGREDIENTS [CABBAGE, CARROT, ONION, RICE, BROCCOLI, CELERY, WATER, SEASONINGS (MODIFIED FOOD STARCH, SOY FLOUR, SUGAR, YEAST EXTRACT, ONION POWDER, MUSHROOM POWDER [MALTODEXTRIN, MUSHROOM, ONION, SALT, SUGAR, YEAST EXTRACT, AND SPICES], SOY SAUCE POWDER [FERMENTED SOYBEANS, WHEAT, SALT AND MALTODEXTRIN], GARLIC POWDER, SALT, BLACK PEPPER, XANTHAN GUM, CAROB BEAN GUM, GUAR GUM]), CRUST INGREDIENTS [ENRICHED FLOUR (WHEAT FLOUR, NIACIN, REDUCED IRON, THIAMINE MONONITRATE, RIBOFLAVIN, FOLIC ACID), WATER, SALT, CORN STARCH, POTATO STARCH, SOY LECITHIN, CULTURED SUGAR, VINEGAR], FRIED IN VEGETABLE OIL), BLANCHED ENRICHED LONG GRAIN PARBOILED RICE (WATER, RICE, IRON, NIACIN, THIAMIN MONONITRATE, FOLIC ACID), WATER, PEAS, CARROTS, RED PEPPERS, HOISIN SAUCE (SUGAR, WATER, SWEET POTATOES, SALT, MODIFIED CORNSTARCH, SOYBEANS, SPICES, SESAME SEEDS, WHEAT FLOUR, GARLIC, CHILI PEPPER, ACETIC ACID), SHERRY WINE, 2% OR LESS OF SUGAR, SOY SAUCE (WATER, WHEAT, SOYBEANS, SALT), ORANGE JUICE CONCENTRATE, MODIFIED CORNSTARCH, WHITE WINE VINEGAR, SOYBEAN OIL, GARLIC PUREE, SESAME OIL, GINGER PUREE (GINGER, WATER, CITRIC ACID), LACTIC ACID, CALCIUM LACTATE.

This one, like most TV Dinners contains yeast extract. Without a flavor enhancer, this frozen concoction would taste bland.

This Banquet TV Dinner also contains MSG.

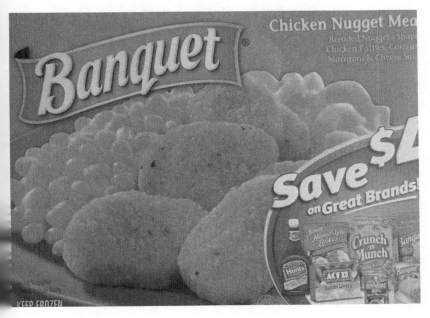

The following gigantic list of stuff contained in this box, including lots of yeast extract, isolated protein, and other chemicals, is necessary to make this dish taste good.

And it works. This dinner tastes good, but it is far from healthy, and it can cause pain and lots of other neurological problems.

INGREDIENTS: COOKED BEER BATTERED CHICKEN PATTY STRIPS (GROUND CHICKEN, ENRICHED FLOUR [WHEAT FLOUR, NIACIN, REDUCED IRON, THIAMINE MONONITRATE, RIBOFLAVIN, FOLIC ACID], WATER, PARTIALLY HYDROGENATED SOYBEAN OIL WITH TBHQ AND CITRIC ACID AS PRESERVATIVES, MODIFIED FOOD STARCH, BEER [WATER, BARLEY, RICE, HOPS, STARCHES, YEAST; CONTAINS WHEAT GLUTEN PROTEIN], SALT, COOKED MASA HARINA [TRACE OF LIME], SOY PROTEIN CONCENTRATE, ISOLATED OAT PRODUCT, SODIUM PHOSPHATE, NATURAL FLAVOR [MALTODEXTRIN, YEAST EXTRACT, NATURAL FLAVOR, POTATO MALTODEXTRIN, SPICES], SODIUM BICARBONATE [HYDROGENATED COTTONSEED OIL], MONOCALCIUM PHOSPHATE [HYDROGENATED COTTONSEED OIL], SPICE, SPICE EXTRACT, ONION POWDER, XANTHAN AND GUAR GUM, DEXTROSE), **ROASTED POTATOES** (ROASTED POTATOES, MALTODEXTRIN, SALT, ONION POWDER, GARLIC POWDER, SPICE, PARSLEY, YEAST EXTRACT, VEGETABLE OIL [SOYBEAN AND SUNFLOWER], DEXTROSE, NATURAL FLAVOR, CARAMEL COLOR, ANNATTO, SODIUM ACID PYROPHOSPHATE), **CHEESE SAUCE** (WATER, CHEESE SAUCE [CHEDDAR CHEESE (MILK, CHEESE CULTURE, SALT, ENZYMES), WATER, MILKFAT, WHEY, ENZYME MODIFIED CHEESE (MILK, WATER, MILKFAT, SODIUM PHOSPHATE, CHEESE CULTURE, SALT, ENZYMES, VITAMIN A PALMITATE), SODIUM PHOSPHATE, MODIFIED FOOD STARCH, SALT, LACTIC ACID, SODIUM ALGINATE, SORBIC ACID AS A PRESERVATIVE, APOCAROTENAL (COLOR)], PASTEURIZED PROCESS CHEDDAR CHEESE [CHEDDAR CHEESE (MILK, CHEESE CULTURE, SALT, ENZYMES), WATER, MILKFAT, ENZYME MODIFIED CHEESE (MILK, WATER, MILKFAT, SODIUM PHOSPHATE, CHEESE CULTURES, SALT, ENZYMES, VITAMIN A PALMITATE), SODIUM PHOSPHATE, SALT, APOCAROTENAL (COLOR)], MODIFIED CORN STARCH, PARTIALLY HYDROGENATED SOYBEAN OIL WITH TBHQ AND CITRIC ACID AS PRESERVATIVES, CHEESE BLEND [CHEDDAR CHEESE, GRANULAR CHEESE, SEMISOFT AND BLUE CHEESE (PASTEURIZED MILK, CHEESE CULTURES, SALT, ENZYMES) WHEY, WATER, SALT, CITRIC ACID), RECONSTITUTED SKIM MILK, SUGAR, SALT, LACTIC ACID, CITRIC ACID, MONO AND DIGLYCERIDES [BHT, CITRIC ACID], SOY PROTEIN CONCENTRATE, DRIED EGG YOLKS, BETA CAROTENE FOR COLOR [CORN OIL, TOCOPHEROL]).

Never eat anything bigger than your head!

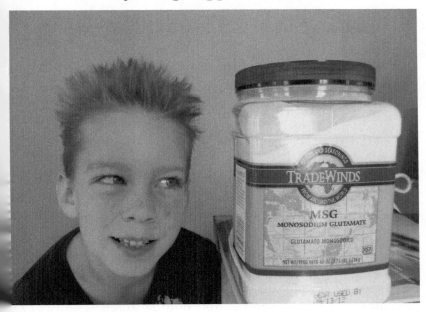

This is a giant jug of MSG and you'll see it in the kitchens of many restaurants.

MSG is toxic to the nervous system, especially to children. The developing nervous systems of young people are highly sus–ceptible to damage by nerve toxins like MSG and aspartame.

Processed foods and candy and chewing gum, fast food, and restaurant food that contain MSG and aspartame and lots of other chemicals are detrimental to the health of kids.

Teenagers and prison inmates have enough angst without exposure to these nerve toxins.

Please don't harm this child, or any child that you care about.

MSG is everywhere, so beware.

Conclusion

Conventional medicine is ineffective for chronic pain.

Conventional medicine fails right from the start, making a wrong turn at the corner of "What did you do?" and "What did you eat?"

"What did you eat?" is not considered. It's never asked.

"What did you do?" is answered and agreed upon very quickly by doctors and patients...if the question comes up at all. And it's a short road that leads from there to the Main Street of modern medicine.

Main Street is lined with orthopedists, neurologists, chiropractors, specialists, physical therapists, massage therapists, acupuncturists, and drug stores ... lots of drug stores.

Main Street dead-ends at the Pain Management Clinic.

The use of drugs, and the very powerful drugs that are injected at the pain management clinics, are dangerous, ineffective, and are often the cause of other problems, including chronic pain.

Doctors know that changing the blood chemistry is a very effective way to decrease inflammation, block pain, and change the human condition in many ways. They change the chemistry by **adding** pharmaceutical agents that unbalance an already unbalanced system.

The system is more effectively balanced by **subtracting**, no adding.

Conventional medicine practitioners are ineffective in curing chronic pain for three reasons:

> They only consider drugs.
>
> They never consider the diet (or the drugs they have prescribed).
>
> They treat pain and chronic pain the same.

Pain and chronic pain are two different things.

Pain is temporary and it heals.

Chronic pain is caused by failure to heal.

Failure to heal is caused by ongoing inflammation.

Ongoing inflammation is caused by substances that are allowed into the blood stream.

Your blood is nourished or poisoned by what enters the body through:

> Inhalation — what you breathe in.
>
> Absorption through the skin (and injections)
>
> Ingestion — what you swallow (diet and drugs)

Chronic pain is due to ongoing inflammation caused by the ongoing ingestion of allergens and/or toxins.

Casein, chocolate, and gluten are the most common allergens.

Toxins are in processed foods and drugs.

Many people who suffer with chronic pain opt for drugs and surgery because they don't know what was discussed in this book.

Some chronic pain sufferers won't find the answers in this book.

Some chronic pain sufferers will not be willing or able to follow these instructions.

Some people must take medication, but only a fraction of those drugs are necessary for very few people.

If you keep going up and down Main Street hoping to find a better doctor or a better drug, you will be disappointed. Main Street should be your last stop.

The approach discussed in this book should be your first move if you suffer with chronic pain.

If that fails, the next approach should be to consider environmental allergens and toxins.

The chemicalization of our food and water and air have caused many health problems.

We are also exposed to soaps, lotions, fabrics, animals, jewelry, shampoos, hair dyes, toothpastes, fluorescent lighting, natural gas appliances, chemically treated furniture, etc.

But our most intimate contact with substances that either nourish us or poison us is what we swallow — diet and drugs.

For chronic pain consider the diet changes and the elimination of drugs first, environmental factors second, and if that fails go to the doctors with their drugs and knives.

Dr. Twogood is available to talk to your group about chronic pain and how to get rid of it.

Contact information:

E-mail: drtwogood@aol.com

Web page: chronicpaingone90days.com

Phone: (760) 953-0861

Address: Dr. Twogood
P.O. Box 3812
Apple Valley, CA 92307

Suggested Reading and Sources

1. Selye, Hans *The Stress of Life*, McGraw-Hill, Inc. 1984

2. Oster, M.D., Kurt and Ross, Ph.D., Donald, *The XO Factor*, Park City Press, New York, 1983

3. Graveline, M.D., Duane, *Statin Drug Side Effects and the Misguided War on Cholesterol*, 2008

4. Oski, M.D., Frank, *Don't Drink Your Milk*, Teach Services, Inc., Brushton, N.Y., 1996

5. Blaylock, M.D., Russell *Excitotoxins, the Taste that Kills*, Health Press, Santa Fe, New Mexico, 1994

6. Rapp, M.D., Doris *Is This Your Child?* William Morrow and Company Inc., New York, 1991

7. Foreman, Robert, *How to Control Your Allergies*, Larchmont Books, Atlanta, Georgia, 1984

8. McDougall, M.D. John
   Read any of his books.

CPSIA information can be obtained at www.ICGtesting.com
Printed in the USA
LVOW012232180613

339232LV00008B/68/P